THERAPY THRO

"This book will do much to sweep away the nonsense and superstition associated with hypnosis. . . . Mr. Rhodes is to be congratulated on the production of a book which will rank as the foremost work of reference, and indeed as a possible classic, for years to come." —*The British Journal of Medical Hypnotism*

THERAPY THROUGH HYPNOSIS explains how hypnotism has been used to cure the mind and the body. Sixteen articles, including interesting and detailed case histories, written by the leading practitioners of hypnotherapy in the United States and in England, describe how hypnotism has cured a variety of psychosomatic ills.

These articles explain what hypnotism is and how it is conducive to rapid psychotherapy, how the use of hypnotism results in cures in a fraction of the time ordinarily required without it. Particular hypnotic techniques, such as the hand levitation method of hypnosis, the induction of hypnogogic reveries, and a technique for overcoming resistance to therapy, are described.

The case histories include a murder-compulsion, a marital problem resulting from unconscious mother-hatred, an hysterical somnambulist with latent homosexual and sadistic tendencies, and many others.

The book also contains an article on Self-Taught Autohypnosis for Insomnia and Obesity, which for the first time presents this new technique.

Raphael H. Rhodes, the editor, is a consulting psychologist in New York City, and the author of *Hypnosis: Theory, Practice and Application,* which has been widely acclaimed as one of the clearest explanations of the techniques of hypnotism.

By Raphael H. Rhodes

HYPNOSIS: THEORY, PRACTICE AND APPLICATION

THERAPY
THROUGH
HYPNOSIS

EDITED BY
RAPHAEL H. RHODES

Foreword by
MELVIN POWERS

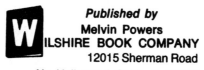

Published by
Melvin Powers
WILSHIRE BOOK COMPANY
12015 Sherman Road
No. Hollywood, California 91605
Telephone: (213) 875-1711 / (818) 983-1105

Printed by

HAL LEIGHTON PRINTING COMPANY
P.O. Box 3952
North Hollywood, California 91605
Telephone: (818) 983-1105

CITADEL PRESS

Designed by Peter A. Dymock

Manufactured in the United States of America

ISBN 0-87980-162-X

In memory of

DR. FOSTER KENNEDY

who strove for the Light;
and for his striving,
was given the Victory as well.

—

FOREWORD

This book will come as a surprise to many laymen who are still confused about the role hypnosis plays in modern medicine. Their surprise will be doubled when they find it was originally published in 1952, and that physicians even then had been using hypnosis successfully in all the specialties for some time.

To those of us who have been part of the modern renaissance in hypnotherapy, it is astonishing to discover how many otherwise well-informed individuals today know little or nothing about a medical and psychiatric modality which has been steadily growing in scope for two decades.

There is a reason for everything, of course, and the reason in this instance seems to be that hypnosis, no matter how routinely it is used by the medical and psychological professions, still is associated with the black arts in the public mind. This is unfortunate because hypnosis is rendering a service possible with no other healing modality.

Considering this knowledge gap by a large segment of the public, it is apparent to me that *Therapy Through Hypnosis* is the best possible book the uninformed can read for certainty that hypnosis is being intensively used in all the specialties. The editor, Raphael H. Rhodes, a well-known psychologist, has used the device of presenting papers by leading hypnotherapists in the most prominent of the medical specialties to lend the book versatility as proof that there is no mystery about the use of hypnosis among prominent therapists.

Mr. Rhodes himself takes on the task of relating what modern hypnosis is and what it does, no small matter considering the misconceptions that are still unbelievably prevalent. With this out of the way, he goes on to recount several revealing case histories from his own practice.

It is difficult to decide which are the most fascinating chapters in this extraordinary volume. You may be surprised, at the very outset, that your tastes, indeed your whole personality, can be changed by hypnotherapy. Dr. Lewis R. Wolberg, a pioneer in the field, contributes the chapter on reconditioning, and it is meticulously drawn.

Mr. Rhodes has included many histories from Dr. Wolberg's case book, and the latter's methods of inducing hypnosis and therapeutic results will be of interest both to laymen and other hypnotherapists. He is one of the few psychiatrists using hypnoanalysis, that is, reducing the long time needed for psychotherapy by the judicious utilization of hypnosis.

Women in particular will be interested in the chapter on obstetrics by Drs. Milton Abramson and William T. Heron, to say nothing of the chapter on gynecologic disorders by Dr. William S. Kroger. Hypnosis for childbirth is probably the best-known use of hypnotherapy, but most readers will be astounded to learn that many "organic" gynecologic symptoms are actually not organic at all but psychosomatic in nature—activated by the mind and self-given suggestion.

Dr. Kroger relates many examples of gynecologic pains that stem from the mind, not the body, and most women, I think, will agree that some of their "female problems" may be due mostly to their inability to be females.

The most lucid and reasoned paper on alcoholism I have ever read has been included, and Dr. S. J. Van Pelt, a British author, offers hope for every family that has a member in the toils of alcohol. Hypnosis, when properly used, can help cure alcoholics.

Dr. Van Pelt's logic is much more persuasive and believable than of many other approaches to alcoholism including Alcoholics Anonymous, Antabuse and the proverbial "bolt from the blue" in which the more hysterical patients are suddenly cured forever by religious commitments.

As I have said, this book can prove of great help to laymen unacquainted with the many uses of hypnosis, but it can prove of almost equal value to the professional healer who has been subjected to a systematic campaign of fear concerning the use of this valuable tool. He has been frightened by the very organization that legitimatized hypnosis in 1958.

This is not the first resurgence of hypnosis. It has been around for thousands of years, and periodically appears in the healing arts, only to die an ignominious death after varying lengths of time, usually after incurring the wrath of doctors who were inept in its use.

I suspect this fairly frequent demise of a proven medical and psychologic aid is always due to a lack of proficiency in its use by the very ones who need it most, but I also suspect this will happen so long as it produces "magical" results and shortens treatment time.

I will go further and say the shortage of doctors is planned, and any mode of treatment that results in quick amelioration of symptoms will always meet with hostility. The psychoanalyst, for instance, wants no modality that reduces the time he now spends with a patient. He firmly believes that every moment spent with the patient is necessary, and seriously (and honestly) is convinced that any abbreviation of his treatment will have an adverse effect on the patient.

All the many present methods of psychotherapy are now

threatened by such treatments as *Psycho-Cybernetics,*[1] applied human cybernetics and other innovative techniques, and most doctors wish to maintain the *status quo.* It is to be hoped that this time hypnosis will retain its rightful place in medicine and not be pushed down by those who seek no progress.

Returning now to Mr. Rhodes' book, I would like to commend him for some of his inclusions. Very few books contain a chapter on hypnosis for children, but in this book there is a bounteous one by Dr. Gordon Ambrose.

It may be said here that children make the best subjects (the optimum age is seven), and treatment at that time may save them from a lifetime of trouble. It is to be hoped that the paper by Dr. Ambrose will lead many parents to seek therapy for their children before the disorder becomes a deep-seated habit of conditioned reflex.

Probably one of the most important chapters in this speeded-up age is the one by Dr. Jacob M. Conn on relaxation. Our age has been rightly called (and the sale of tranquilizers proves it) the age of anxiety, and Dr. Conn convincingly tells how we can remain calm in the midst of turmoil.

So tense and anxious have we become, that "keyed-up executives" has become a by-phrase of everyday life. Dr. Conn has much to say about how one can remain placid without becoming bovine.

There are many more important chapters in this remarkable book which I think is one of the best on hypnosis and its uses I have ever read. But read them for yourself. You will be astounded at some of the uses of this age-old therapy.

My intention has been to whet your appetite for the feast to come, and I devoutly hope I have succeeded. At any rate, you will be a wiser individual when you reach the last page.

(1) *Psycho-Cybernetics,* Maxwell Maltz, M.D., Hollywood, California 90069, Wilshire Book Company, 1963

I hope you will concentrate on the many fine chapters. They can change all your ideas about hypnosis, a medical modality that has never received the attention it deserved.

It is my belief this book will afford you the most informative reading on hypnosis you have ever encountered.

Persevere in your efforts to learn the extent of modern hypnosis, and accept my best wishes in your efforts.

Melvin Powers

12015 Sherman Road
No. Hollywood, California 91605

PREFACE

The average man does not understand hypnosis. His concept of it is formed from a hodgepodge of fact and fancy. At best, he has witnessed a stage demonstration of hypnotic domination, the genuineness of which he probably questions. But whether he regards hypnotism as something obscure, or whether he suspects it of being supernatural or even fraudulent, at any rate, he is sure that it has no relationship to his own life and problems.

This misconception of what hypnosis is, this lack of appreciation of what it can do and how it can help him, is due in part to the fact that most serious writing about hypnotism is in scientific language, and that practically all of it is published in technical books or scientific journals which the average man never reads.

I have attempted to cull here some of the authoritative writings in the field of hypnotism, choosing material which appeared to me to be simple in style and interesting in content so that the general reader, as well as the specialist, might read the collection with pleasure and profit. In selecting and editing this material, my purpose has been to introduce hypnotism to those who have not understood it before, and to acquaint them with its power to alleviate and cure many types of mental distress and functional physical disturbances and disorders.

With this purpose in view I have bypassed the technical writings pertaining to hypnotic theory, technique, and experimental investigation. The interested scientist will find them elsewhere. But he who asks, "Can hypnotism help me?" may find his answer here.

This volume should prove of value also to practitioners of

hypnotherapy. A large part of the selected material consists of case histories, including verbatim questions and answers. This type of presentation specifically illustrates many of the devices and methods used for therapy through hypnosis.

RAPHAEL H. RHODES

ACKNOWLEDGMENTS

I am grateful to the authors of the articles in this volume for their contributions, and to their publishers and editors who have consented to the reprinting of copyrighted material.

The full list of credits pertaining to each article is detailed under Notes and References.

I also wish to express my appreciation for the invaluable editorial advice and assistance of Irma G. Rhodes.

R.H.R.

CONTENTS

CONTENTS

HYPNOSIS:

WHAT IT IS AND WHAT IT DOES

BY

RAPHAEL H. RHODES

———————————

Hypnotism is a scientific psychological tool. When properly used, it is the safest means of curing many types of mental distress in the shortest possible time. Hypnosis cuts down the time required for ordinary psychoanalysis to a fraction of the usual length of treatment. Used together with psychoanalysis, hypnosis often results in cures in less than one-tenth of the time necessary without it.

Hypnosis is absolutely safe. There is no case on record reporting harmful results from its therapeutic use. In this respect it has a clear advantage over electric shock therapy or brain surgery, which may sometimes result in serious impairment of memory or loss of mental function. Hypnotism never harms the memory; rather, it strengthens it. Hypnosis achieves its results, not by destroying mental channels, but by reclaiming them.

When one's acquaintance with hypnotism is limited to what he has seen on the stage, his ideas about it are probably quite wrong. The public entertainer is interested in laughs, and when he employs hypnotism, he gets his laughs by making his subjects look and act like puppets. The audience sometimes gets the impression that the hypnotist has some magic power. He may explain that hypnotic control is scientific rather than supernatural. Yet, the nature of his performance makes it seem that a hypnotized person is simply a weak-willed automaton, completely dominated by a master-mind.

That impression is wholly erroneous. It results from an incomplete and one-sided presentation of the subject. Hypnotism is a psychological phenomenon of profound value in mental therapy. Moreover, when its use for this purpose is understood, hypnotism proves even more fascinating than when presented merely for the amusement of an audience.

Before one can understand what hypnotism can do, he must know what it is. Hypnosis is a state of mind. It is a passive state of mind, akin to ordinary sleep. Like sleep, it is a state of mind in which the driving conscious thoughts of the waking hours have been put aside. This leaves the mental arena clear for the uninhibited sway of subconscious thought. Once the active preoccupations of waking consciousness have been temporarily cast aside, the subconscious factors of the mind rise to the threshold of thought. As in sleep, the conscious mind recedes, and the subconscious mind is in control.

There is, however, an important difference between hypnosis and sleep. In ordinary sleep the conscious mind withdraws and the subconscious comes to the fore without outside direction. In hypnosis, it is the hypnotist who forces the mental shift, and the subconscious mind comes to the fore subject to the hypnotist's control, and ready to follow any suggestions he may make to it.[1]

Thus, once the hypnotist has brought about the mental shift, he controls the subject's subconscious mind. He can make suggestions to it, and these will be carried out. Often even after the subject is awake, he will follow suggestions made to him during the hypnotic trance. This is called posthypnotic suggestion.

It also happens that memory is lodged in the subconscious. Consequently, while a person is in the hypnotic state, his memory is better than in his waking state. Things which he could not recall while awake, are easily remembered in hypnotic trance. Thus the hypnotist can force his subject to recall and reveal long forgotten incidents and buried memories. This is particularly important in psychological therapy.

Mental distress is frequently the result of memories which are buried in the subconscious. Incidents or thoughts of an unpleasant or shocking nature were suppressed, and became lodged in the subconscious mind. They are forgotten, as far as the conscious mind is concerned. But they persist in the subconscious and, without the individual's being aware of it, they affect his thought pattern. Such buried memories often cause severe mental anguish. In some cases they may even produce an apparently physical disorder, although there is actually no organic defect.

In all such cases, a cure is possible only if these subconscious incidents and memories are first brought back to the realm of conscious thought and reevaluated. In every such case hypnotism, which brings the subconscious to the fore, can quickly and effectively open the gate that barred the mind from freedom.

THE DYNAMICS OF MURDER

Take the case of Mrs. B., for example. When she first called upon me, she said she was desperate. For the past four years she had had a compulsion to murder people—anyone; her husband, friends, strangers—everyone. It was getting worse all the time. The first time she felt the drive, she was in a motion picture theatre. She suddenly remembered she had a hatchet at home. When she got home, she took the hatchet, walked with it to a brook, and threw it away.

But the desire to kill persisted. When she saw a knife or a blunt object, she wanted to use it on anyone who was near her. During the first year this happened only occasionally, maybe once a month or so. But then the desire became stronger and more frequent. She fought against it. She felt she really did not hate anyone and did not want to harm anyone, but the fearful compulsion came upon her more and more; more strongly and more often. Finally it was with her almost all the time. She began to avoid her friends, hoping to conquer the monster by self-imposed seclusion. It did not help. She even began to feel the same way toward her husband, although she really loved him.

"Sometimes he's in the kitchen and I'm drying a pot, and holding it by the handle, and I feel as if I want to hit him on the head with it and kill him—and I just stop myself in time, and the next minute I want to take him in my arms and kiss him," she said. "I worship him, and the thought that I might hurt him drives me crazy. I'm even afraid to ride on the subway, because I get the urge to push people off the platform in front of the train. Why is that? I don't even know the people. I'm so afraid. If you don't help me, I don't know what I'll do. Perhaps I'll kill myself. I've wanted to do that too."

I hypnotized her and said, "Your mind will now go back to the first time you had this desire to kill someone. Was there any such time before the hatchet incident?" She answered, "I once wanted to kill my mother." "When was that?" "About a year before my marriage, just after we'd become engaged. I was nailing a rug down and my mother was standing there, and suddenly I had the desire to hit her on the head with the hammer. I had forgotten that. I loved my mother very much."

Her father had died when she was very young, and she had been reared by her mother. She had lived with her mother until her marriage at age thirty, about five years before she came to seek treatment. Her mother had died about six months after the marriage. There were no children. "I've been afraid to have a child, because I thought I might kill it," she said.

Before awakening her from the hypnotic trance, I said, "Between today and the next time you come here, you will have a dream which will symbolize the cause of your difficulty, and you will remember that dream and the next time you come here you will report it to me."

At the next session she said, "I had a nightmare last night. I dreamed I was driving my car down a steep hill. I was alone in it. At the bottom of the hill were the railroad tracks, and the gate was closed and a train was coming. The brakes were bad and I tried very hard and finally I stopped the car. And then I saw another car coming down the hill, and there were three men in it, and they were talking and laughing. They didn't pay any attention to the train, and I kept yelling, 'No, No, No,' but they didn't listen and they went right on downhill and through the gate, and Oh! my, they were all killed. And I just got out of the car and said, 'No, it isn't so,' but I could see a head here and an arm there. It was terrible, and I woke up, and couldn't fall asleep any more. But I don't see what that has to do with my case."

My questions and her answers, in summary, follow:

Q. Do the men in the dream remind you of anyone you know?

A. No.

Q. Does your driving downhill make you think of anything?

A. No. Except that I'm so awfully afraid all the time.

Q. What are you afraid of?

A. I don't know. I'm always afraid. I'm afraid something will happen to me.

Q. What may happen to you?

A. I don't know. But I feel it's something terrible. People are going to do something to me.

Q. Who were the men in the car?

A. I didn't recognize any of them. There have been many men in my life. Before I got married, I led a loose life, went with anyone who wanted me. I didn't think anything of it. My mother was the same way and it used to seem all right. I was flattered if any man paid attention to me. But, you know, even before I got married, I changed. I'd look at men who were dressed nicely coming off a train, and I'd think, "I wish some decent guy like that would marry me." And then when I met my husband, he didn't know about my past, and he is such a fine man, I couldn't ever tell him about it, and, of course, I've been absolutely faithful to him.

Q. Are you happy with your husband?

A. Very happy. My life would be perfect if I didn't have this constant desire to kill people.

Q. Did you want to kill the men in the car?

A. I don't think so. I kept shouting, "No, No, No," but they didn't listen to me.

Q. Describe the men you saw in the car.

A. Well, one of them—I keep thinking of the word *esthetic*. That's the type I used to like. He was tall, thin, had delicate features. He was just like one fellow I used to know.

Q. And the others?

A. They were the same type.

Q. Anyone in particular?

A. I don't think so. But they were the same type as the men I used to go for. Do you think I really wanted them to be killed?

Q. What do you think?

A. I'm not sure. I wonder if I should tell my husband about my past. I don't like to keep it secret from him.

Q. Why not?

A. If he ever found out, he might leave me and that would kill me. He's my whole life.

Q. Did the men in the dream represent the type of people who share this secret you are keeping from your husband?

A. Yes. I never thought of that before. Did I really want to kill them? I like people. I don't want anybody to die.

Q. If all the people who know about your past were suddenly killed by an atom bomb—you had nothing to do with it, and didn't know about it until afterwards—but they were all wiped off the earth by an atom bomb, would you be happy?

A. I—I guess, yes, I might. Yes, I would.

Subsequent discussion clarified the details. Her first impulse to kill, directed against the mother who had fostered her loose ways, came upon her just after her engagement. Her mother knew the secret she was keeping from her fiance. Her mother might reveal it and this was a threat to her happiness. After her marriage, other people who shared the secret represented a similar threat to her new way of life. She wished them dead. But, being fundamentally a decent, sensitive and conscientious person, she suppressed these thoughts, forcibly and completely. They lodged in her subconscious. Then, without her being aware of their source, they manifested themselves in the form of a compulsion to murder at random.

This compulsive drive was directed not only against the men who shared her secret; it was directed also against all people, society in general, based upon a subconscious feeling of being misunderstood. It was directed even against her husband, who, again subconsciously, was a major factor in her problem.

Ultimately she decided to tell her husband everything. "I think it's worth the risk. I can't go on this way," she said. So she unburdened her secret to him. When the secret became nonexistent, her compulsive drives disappeared.

The use of hypnotism in this case forced a quick revelation of the underlying problem and resulted in a rapid cure. The increased memory of the subject under hypnosis made possible an almost immediate recall of the first time she had experienced this desire to kill someone. The posthypnotic suggestion of a relevant dream raised the deeply buried subconscious memories and desires to the threshold of consciousness. Here they were readily understood and reevaluated in a normal way. Once they assumed their normal place in the sphere of thought, the cure was assured.

THE QUEST FOR NORMALCY

Several different techniques were used in the case of Mr. Q. He was thirty years of age, held a well-paying job, and appeared to be a normal and likeable fellow. But he was afraid to get married, although he desired to have a wife and children. "I'm afraid I'm a homosexual," he said. "I've never had any relations with women, and ever since my high school days I've had a desire to fondle men. I haven't ever done it, but I've wanted to so many times. I think there's something wrong with me. Can you help me?"

Q. When did you first have this desire?

A. In high school. I liked to play baseball, and I finally made the school team. Then I felt this desire for the other boys on the team. Not only them, but others too.

Q. Did you ever speak to anyone about it?

A. No. Never did anything either. But I always wanted to. Sometimes I still want to. Of course, I stay away from people now and keep to myself as much as possible. I'm afraid if I get too friendly with a man, I might try to do something wrong.

Q. How about women?

A. I'm afraid to go with them. I'd like to get married and have a family, but if there's this thing wrong with me, I wouldn't make a good husband.

During the course of this and subsequent sessions, Mr. Q. reported that he had come from a poor home, was often undernourished as a child, and had fainted from hunger in elementary school. That was when he was about eight years old. His classmates had taunted him, called him "weak fish" and "sissy." He resented their insults and withdrew from them, but at the same time he craved their friendship. This resulted in a vicious circle of frustration. Although he longed for the companionship of his young friends, he was afraid to join in their sports because he might display some weakness which they would ridicule. The more he withdrew from them, the more they jeered at him; the more they jeered at him, the more he withdrew. The result was that he got less and less of the comradeship he wanted most, and considered himself an outcast. This was the emotional environment which conditioned most of his elementary school and early high school life.

And then he became conscious of those desires which made his feelings of withdrawal and loneliness complete.

I put him into a trance, and suggested that between this session and the next one he would have a dream which would help him recall how his homosexual impulses had started. At the next session Mr. Q. reported that he had had a dream about a hike in the country. He went along with a number of the boys from his neighborhood. They took their lunch, and stayed all day. The boys didn't play with him because he was a weakling. That is all he could remember.

Q. What were the names of some of these boys?

A. I remember one. His name was Jonathan.

Q. Did you dream anything else about Jonathan?

A. There was nothing else in the dream. But now I recall an incident that happened before that, with Jonathan. The kids on the block were playing ball and I wanted to join the game, but one fellow who was a big bully said, "Go away, we don't want sissies," and I was so hurt I couldn't say anything, and I just sat down on the curb. And then this kid, Jonathan, came over and said something nice to me, and I felt awfully good about it. It meant a lot to me.

Q. Did you become friendly with Jonathan?

A. I suppose it didn't mean too much to him; he probably didn't think about it. But after that I felt he was my friend. Anyway I knew he wouldn't tease me. And after that I felt good when he was around. But as I think back now, he didn't seem to care one way or the other.

Q. Didn't the dream have anything particular about Jonathan in it?

A. I don't think so. I can't remember.

At this point I used two more hypnotic techniques. One is called crystal gazing and the other is known as automatic writing. I put

Mr. Q. into hypnotic trance, and said, "When I snap my fingers, you will open your eyes but remain asleep. You will look into this crystal ball. You will see an image which will recall to you what part Jonathan played in the dream, and you will tell it to me."

When Mr. Q. opened his eyes and looked at the crystal ball, he said, "I see Jonathan and another boy. They are lying on the grass. They are fondling each other and laughing."

Q. Stay asleep, and answer my questions. Did that actually ever happen?

A. Yes. I remember it now. It happened on that hike. I saw it and was disgusted and turned away. I have never thought of it since then.

Q. What does fondling between men mean to you? Why do you want to do it?

A. I don't know.

Q. Take this pencil in your right hand. I'm holding a pad for you. When I say, *write,* your hand will write something on the pad which will explain why you want to fondle men. Now, *write* while I hold the pad.

He scrawled the word *friendship.* I said, "When you wake up, you'll remember everything that happened while you were asleep. Now, when I count to ten, you'll wake up."

The discussion which followed synthesized Mr. Q.'s past with his present. As a child, he had longed for the friendship of his boyhood companions. This desire was frustrated. After Jonathan had shown him the single act of kindness, which to him assumed momentous significance, he desired friendship with Jonathan most of all. When he saw the actions of Jonathan and the other boy on the hike, he thought that such behavior must be an expression of friendship between them, yet he was consciously disgusted and turned away. He even "forgot" the incident. But the subconscious never forgets.

The memory of that incident lodged in his subconscious mind. Forcefully rejected by his conscious mind, it had lodged in his subconscious in its original unanalyzed form, coupled only with the thought that he desired friendship with Jonathan. The desire for friendship, and the buried memory of the actions he had witnessed, had become interwoven and interrelated subconsciously. Jonathan and the other boy were friends; they had fondled each other; fondling represented friendship. So the unanalytical subconscious had received it, and so it had remained embedded there those many years.

The abnormal concept had manifested itself as an abnormal desire. Until he understood its origin, he had had no way of successfully combatting it, and so he had remained its slave. As soon as he understood it consciously, and was able to reevaluate it logically, its impact and power were destroyed, and the abnormal desire disappeared. "It all seems so foolish now," he said.

Here again hypnotism made possible the use of special techniques for quickly probing the subconscious, thereby saving many months or perhaps even years of searching which might have been required with analysis alone. The techniques of memory recall, dream induction, crystal gazing, and automatic writing are only a few of the psychological tools made possible by hypnotism. Some of the others are known as experimentally induced disorder, age regression, dream recall, and symptom alleviation. They may be used singly or in appropriate combination. In every case they will foster rapid recall and reevaluation of the crucial incidents underlying a mental disorder.

THE POWER OF SUGGESTION

In some cases, worthwhile results may be achieved by the use of posthypnotic suggestion alone without analysis. Mr. A. was asked to make a speech at a political rally. He was anxious to make a good impression. He had prepared his talk thoroughly, knew just what he wanted to say. Still now, a few hours before delivery time, he was as nervous as a soldier before his first real battle. He could hardly control his trembling.

I put him into a light trance. While he slept, I suggested that he would become calm and relaxed, that after he awoke, he would remain calm and relaxed; that he would think clearly and easily, and that the words of his speech would come to him without difficulty; finally, that he would deliver the speech fearlessly and convincingly. When awakened, he remained calm and relaxed, and the next day he telephoned to report that his speech had been successful beyond all expectations.

Posthypnotic suggestion, with or without analysis, is a powerful psychological device. It may be helpful in many types of complaint including insomnia, disturbing dreams, various fears and phobias, nervous headache, nervous habits such as nail-biting, excessive smoking, intemperate eating or drinking, functional speech disorders, and personality defects such as shyness, pugnacity, temper, awkwardness, dependency, and so forth.

SAVINGS IN TIME AND MONEY

A few years ago the United States Social Security Board estimated that about 8,000,000 U.S. citizens were neurotic. The figures were based largely on Selective Service statistics. *Time* magazine,[2] which reported the findings, added that analysts' fees for treatment range from $5.00 to $50.00 an hour; that "the average treatment (an hour a day, five days a week) takes 18 months," and costs between $1,500.00 and $5,000.00. Apparently hypnotism was not employed in those sessions.

With the aid of hypnotism, Mrs. B., who had had the compulsion to murder, was cured in a total of seven sessions. Before trying hypnoanalysis, she had been seeing an analyst for two years with indifferent results. Mr. Q. had never consulted any other psychologist, but it is reasonable to assume that without the use of the hypnotic techniques of dream induction, crystal gazing, and automatic writing, his buried memories might well have taken many months, perhaps longer, to come to the surface in free association alone. The use of hypnotism in his case made possible the achievement of a cure in eight sessions.

Within the past decade or two hypnosis has been employed on an everincreasing scale by psychiatrists and psychologists for the relief and cure of psychic disturbances and nonorganic disorders. The Menninger Clinic in Topeka, Kansas, The Johns Hopkins Hospital in Baltimore, Maryland, the Wayne County Hospital in Eloise, Michigan, and the Psychiatric Division of Bellevue Hospital in New York, New York, are a few of the many institutions throughout the country at which the extensive use and successful application of hypnotism have been recorded.

Nevertheless, popular misconceptions about the subject still persist, reflected in the wide variety of attitudes towards it. They range from unreasoning rejection to unreasoning acceptance of everything ever imputed to the powers of hypnotism. The elusive truth, as so often happens, lies along some middle ground.

The subconscious, in which the origins of neuroses are concealed, is resistant to conscious probing. Hypnotism is a scientific key which opens the ivory gate of the abode of sleep and thus facilitates a return to the hidden past. It is a useful instrument for the reexamination of the past and the reorientation of the present. It is the surest aid to rapid psychotherapy.

HYPNOSIS IN RECONDITIONING

BY

LEWIS R. WOLBERG, M.D.

The fact that neurotic patterns of behavior are the product of faulty conditionings suggests that normal behavior patterns may be substituted by a process of reconditioning.

Among the earliest work along this line is that of Jones[1] who experimented with a child who had been bitten by a rabbit, and had developed great fear of the animal and of rabbits in general. Jones believed that if he could get the child to associate the rabbit with a pleasant emotion, fear of the creature might be lost. He decided to feed the child appetizing foods when the latter became hungry, at the same time exposing the child to the sight of the rabbit held at a distance; then gradually diminishing the distance. The experiment was successful and the child no longer experienced fear of the rabbit.

Other reconditioning experiments have been performed by Yates,[2] Max[3] and Mowrer and Mowrer.[4] Yates, treating a girl who was upset emotionally by the presence of men, had her repeat the word "calm," associating to it ideas of security, well-being, and peace. She gradually learned that constant repetition of the word in the presence of men sufficed to maintain her emotional composure. Max treated a homosexual patient who was obsessed with homosexual thoughts whenever he came in contact with a certain inanimate object. Presenting this object to the patient at the same time he was given an electric shock sufficed to terminate the power of the object to excite homosexual thoughts. Mowrer and Mowrer treated enuresis by constructing an apparatus that was placed in the bed of the enuritic child, which when wet caused a circuit to close and to ring a bell, awakening the child. They discovered that after three or four such experiences, the impulse alone to urinate aroused the child.

All of these experiments are dependent upon reconditioning the individual to painful or pleasurable stimuli. Because hypnosis is capable of intensifying emotional stimuli, and because it renders the patient more susceptible to the establishing of conditional reflexes,[5, 6] it would seem to lend itself admirably to this therapeutic technic.

An example of how reconditioning is effected under hypnosis may be illustrated by the case of a woman who had, since childhood, experienced an intense dislike for orange juice which gradually had extended itself to other citrus fruits. Even the sight of an orange nauseated her, and on several occasions she had to leave the dinner table when this fruit was served. Her reaction caused her great social embarrassment. She associated her dislike with the fact that her mother had forced her, during childhood, to drink castor oil which had been mixed with orange juice. Indeed, whenever she tasted a citrus juice, she imagined she was imbibing castor oil.

Treatment consisted of discussing with her the mechanism of conditioning in relation to her own experience. Under hypnosis she was asked to dream about the happiest and most enjoyable episodes in her life. She was enjoined to fantasy the most pleasurable experiences that might happen to a person. Then a suggestion was given her that she would feel unbounded happiness and pleasure in the trance, as if the experiences were happening all over again or as if she were fulfilling her fantasies. As soon as she responded to these suggestions, she was asked to imagine herself in an orange grove while enjoying the same emotional state. Suggestions were then made that she would lose her dislike for fruit juice because the dislike would be replaced by pleasure. Indeed she would, to her surprise, find herself wanting to drink orange juice because she realized she did not dislike it as much as she had imagined. A sip of diluted orange juice was given her and she admitted that it produced no nausea.

During later sessions, these suggestions were repeated, and she was given stronger and stronger concentrations of citrus juices. When she was capable of drinking undiluted orange juice, a post-hypnotic suggestion was made to the effect that she would be able in the waking state to drink fruit juices of all types, and to look at fruits with enjoyment instead of disgust. Those suggestions were successful and the patient overcame her phobia.

Phobias that have been established on the basis of fortuitous conditionings are most easily influenced by this technic. Habits which the patient finds difficult to break, such as excessive smoking, nail-biting, eating, and alcoholic indulgence, and some forms of drug addiction respond very well to this method. The aim is to replace the pleasure feelings associated with these habits with disagreeable emotions, in the effort to get the patient to abandon his habit.

In the trance state the patient is told that he will experience less and less of a desire to indulge his habit, and its control will contribute to his self-respect and feelings of happiness. Painful or disgusting experiences in the life of the individual, and fantasies of a disagreeable nature which he brings up in the trance, are linked to his craving. When an association is established in the patient's mind, the conditioning process is tested by permitting him to indulge his habit in hypnosis. For instance, in an alcoholic patient, nausea and vomiting may be associated to the drinking of alcohol, and success in the conditioning process is achieved when the patient disgorges a drink he is encouraged to imbibe. Following the successful establishing of the conditioned reflex, posthypnotic suggestions are made along the same line. The patient will require regular reinforcement of these suggestions for a considerable period thereafter.

In some instances, it may be possible to condition an individual to react comfortably to interpersonal situations to which he customarily responds with tension and discomfort. For example, a patient, who lived out of town and could spend only a few weeks in therapy, complained that when he was in the presence of other people, he was intensely disturbed and uncomfortable. In the trance it was determined that he felt competitive with others and anticipated criticism and attack. Feelings of relaxation were induced by suggesting a peaceful isolated scene on the seashore. Then in fantasy a person was introduced. The patient was urged to maintain his tranquility by thinking and talking about those subjects with which he was most conversant, avoiding controversial topics. The pleasurable emotional tone persisted until the patient found himself engaging in a fantasied argument with his companion. By shifting the conversation, he again relaxed. Gradually, more and more people were introduced in the scene, and the patient was able to appreciate quite vividly how his tranquility was upset by his own attitudes. He was able to transfer to the waking state what he had learned in the trance. In a group he experienced the same feelings of comfort and relaxation, and he was able to maintain his tranquility by choosing and concentrating on the more pleasurable aspects of the situation.

Success in reconditioning is possible only where the symptom or habit does not serve a vitally dynamic purpose in the life adjustment of the individual. Where a symptom has a deep symbolic value, particularly as a defense against anxiety, reconditioning suggestions will usually be unsuccessful until the patient has achieved emotional insight.

In phobias of anxiety hysteria, for instance, exposing the patient to the phobic situation while undergoing an artificially imposed state of happiness or ecstasy, may awaken the patient or cause him to condition in an opposite direction, that is, to associate fear with conditions which hitherto had been associated with happiness or ecstasy.

In some instances the patient may seem to respond favorably to an imaginary situation in which he exposes himself to his phobia. An agoraphobic patient in a state of induced ecstasy may, if given a suggestion that he imagines himself outdoors walking around, execute these directions, creating the impression that he has overcome his phobia. However, the patient is quite conscious that he is playing a role, and will willingly go through the motions suggested to him provided he is not actually exposed to his phobia. In the waking state he will still respond with undiminished terror when faced with a real situation. It is important to remember that symptoms usually have an important symbolic significance and that reconditioning may be unsuccessful until the symptom no longer serves a vital function.

A patient with claustrophobia, revealed, through his associations and dreams, that the situation that made him most happy was one in which he was in close contact with his fiancée. He was extremely dependent upon this woman, and when separated from her felt an abysmal loneliness. He was constantly preoccupied with thoughts concerning her whereabouts, and whenever they were apart, he could scarcely wait until they were reunited. His fantasies were concerned with his being embraced or fondled by a maternal woman.

As a child he had been overprotected by a solicitous, domineering mother who had babied and mothered him to excess. He apparently wanted to perpetuate the mother-child relationship in his later contacts with women. Even consciously the thing he wanted most was a love relationship with a woman older than himself. In deep hypnosis this desire was fulfilled in fantasy by suggested dramatized situations in which he was close to an older woman. The patient fairly exuded happiness on suggestions that he was being petted by his fiancée. At the same time a suggestion was given him that he was together with her in an elevator, in the attempt to get him to associate being in a closed place with being embraced by his fiancée. He responded favorably to this while in a trance.

However, in real life his claustrophobia did not vanish. With an analytic technic it was found that this symptom was in part the result of a feeling that he was trapped and might suffer mutilation in a close contact with a woman. Only after his relationship with women straightened out to a point where he felt he did not have to violate his independence or freedom in closeness, was it possible to recondition him successfully.

ILLUSTRATIVE CASE

The following case illustrates the use of hypnosis with a directive, persuasive and reeducational approach. The symptom for which the patient sought help was premature ejaculation which was so severe that intercourse was impossible. A transcription of the entire treatment (which consisted of eight sessions over a period of a little more than one month) follows.

First Session (April 1)

The patient presents his problem which is premature ejaculation, so severe that complete penetration is impossible. His moti-

*vation for therapy is a desire for a normal sex life. Responses to
the Rorschach cards and Goodenough test indicate severe neurotic
problems. However, he sees no difficulty in any other area of psychobiologic functioning than the sexual one. There is no desire
on his part to inquire into his interpersonal relationships and for
this reason a directive approach is decided on at the start.*

Pt. I have been suffering for many years, Doctor, of what I
believe is premature ejaculation. It is an outgrowth, I imagine,
from a period of masturbation in childhood. And I put off marriage because that fear was constantly present in my mind. In
going to some sources of books, I happened across Dr. Robinson's
book, who cited cases similar to mine, and whereby he had done
very good work along those lines that were cured. Well, I then
went to see a medical doctor who examined me and said there was
nothing wrong organically, but that as a result of the masturbation, he thought that a certain conditioning was set up which
will be, has to be, overcome. He wasn't very specific as to what
channels I might use, but it was evident that he, as a medical man,
found nothing wrong organically, that he could do nothing
for me.

Dr. I see. How old are you?

Pt. Thirty-six.

Dr. And you are married?

Pt. Married only a short time.

Dr. How long?

Pt. Six weeks.

Dr. And you felt for a long time your condition was hopeless?

Pt. My conviction that it wasn't hopeless dates back about eight
months ago, and when I broached the subject of marriage, to my
doctor, and told him frankly that the fear of being unsuccessful
has kept me from marrying, and truthfully by nature I don't
want to live alone, he said he thought it would be perfectly all
right for me to venture into marriage, feeling certain that I
wouldn't encounter too much difficulty and it would wear off
in time. And I married, as I said, six weeks back.

Dr. Yes.

Pt. Of course I'm trying to regulate myself as much as possible.

I've had a better attitude than when I was single, but not sufficient improvement in performance to be at all successful.

Dr. I see.

Pt. Now I was thinking if as the doctor had mentioned that there was nothing organically wrong, I thought perhaps hypnosis would help. If it is not too extreme conditioning of that habit.

Dr. As you get into the thing and get an idea as to what's behind this premature ejaculation, we can then discuss whether hypnosis is the method of choice. At first I want to ask you just a few more questions. When you married your wife, how long did you know her?

Pt. Oh, about three months.

Dr. How old a woman is she?

Pt. Thirty-four.

Dr. She's never been married?

Pt. No.

Dr. And had she had any relations before?

Pt. No, she hasn't.

Dr. Were you able to penetrate?

Pt. Not fully. Her hymen has not been dilated.

Dr. Are you in love with her?

Pt. Very much.

Dr. Is she understanding?

Pt. Very.

Dr. And patient?

Pt. That's right, very much so.

Dr. What about her own sexual feelings? Is she responsive or cold?

Pt. Yes, she's quite responsive.

Dr. Does she have an orgasm?

Pt. On occasion, she doesn't permit herself to go too far, but on occasion she does when I play with her. See, that's the peculiar thing I might add that might be helpful, that I could play with her until she does reach an orgasm. But the minute I insert, I mean, it happens. I mean the ejaculation comes.

Dr. Yes.

Pt. But it has always been a source of surprise to me that I could hold back indefinitely and have it arise until I try to insert. She is so stimulated sometimes that she has an orgasm and she likes it.

Dr. When she has an orgasm, is it easier for you to control yourself? Or the ejaculation, does it come, none-the-less?

Pt. It comes immediately when I try to insert it.

Dr. I see. Ah, now let us go back a little bit farther. Supposing you tell me about your first relationships with women. How far back do they go?

Pt. Well they go considerably far back. Going up to a prostitute's home on occasion.

Dr. And do you remember the first time?

Pt. Yes.

Dr. What was the occasion? Can you describe it to me?

Pt. Well, if I remember, I think there were three of us, two friends and myself, and we went up to a place in midtown New York. There were three rather attractive girls. I think the experience was the same even at the first time, if I remember correctly. I think the ejaculation came very fast there, too. The girl was nice; there wasn't anything repulsive about it as I remember her. But the experience has been in that way, and it's been that way ever since more or less.

Dr. Now, supposing we go back now into your early childhood. Start in with your parents. Are your parents alive?

Pt. My mother is, my dad passed away a short time ago.

Dr. What sort of person is she?

Pt. Well, very fine, very homelike. The family spirit has been very fine all through the years. The feeling of devotion and loyalty between members and between parent and children, it's been a high type.

Dr. And what about your relationship with you mother, What sort of a relationship was it?

Pt. Well. . . .

Dr. Were you attached to her, were you very fond of her, or were you detached?

Pt. No, normally fond. We always had a high regard not only for mother, but for father and mother I mean.

Dr. Did she domineer you?

Pt. No.

Dr. You could do pretty much as you wanted?

Pt. That's right.

Dr. And what sort of a person was your father?

Pt. Very much the same. He was of a religious nature.

Dr. Was he a domineering person?

Pt. No.

Dr. Restrictive, repressive?

Pt. Not restrictive, no. He was liberal minded.

Dr. And you loved him?

Pt. That's right.

Dr. Did you prefer your mother or your father?

Pt. No, it was about equal there. There was no preference for either of them.

Dr. And what about your brothers and sisters?

Pt. I have no brothers; I have three sisters, older than myself.

Dr. And their personalities are what?

Pt. They're very much like my own.

Dr. How do you get along with them?

Pt. Very well indeed.

Dr. How would you describe your own personality?

Pt. Well, it's difficult to define.

Dr. For instance, how do you get along with people?

Pt. Very well, very well.

Dr. Do you get along on submissive or domineering lines?

Pt. No, just the middle type.

Dr. You can hold your own with people.

Pt. Definitely, socially and in business. I am in charge of several people.

Dr. Are you able to adopt a leadership role?

Pt. Definitely I am; I have no difficulty along those lines.

Dr. Do you get at all hostile towards people?

Pt. No.

Dr. Now what about symptoms? Do you get any depressive symptoms of any kind?

Pt. No.

Dr. Any anxiety?

Pt. No.

Dr. Do you have any phobias of any kind?

Pt. No.

Dr.   Any fears, any obsessions of any kind?

Pt.   No.

Dr.   Do you feel compelled to do certain things?

Pt.   No, no.

Dr.   Any headaches or stomach trouble or other physical complaints?

Pt.   No.

Dr.   Do you feel tense? Emotionally tense?

Pt.   Occasionally, yes; emotionally, no.

Dr.   Any insomnia?

Pt.   No.

Dr.   Any nightmares?

Pt.   No.

Dr.   Alcoholism?

Pt.   No.

Dr.   Sedatives?

Pt.   No.

Dr.   How about dreams? Do you dream?

Pt.   Well I have not for the longest time; I never did, ah, often. It's a rarity with me.

Dr.   You weren't a nervous child?

Pt.   No.

Dr.   Do you remember any dreams you have had at all?

Pt.   No, I really couldn't say. I really couldn't say.

Dr.   Do you recall any repetitive dreams as a child?

Pt.   No.

(Up to this point in the interview it would seem that the patient has no problems other than the symptom of premature ejaculation. He is not aware of any difficulties in interpersonal relations.)

Dr.   All right, I'm going to show you some cards of ink blots, and I'd like to have you look at these and tell me what comes to your mind. It's not really a test, merely impressions as to what may be going on in your deeper emotional life.

Pt.   I see.

Dr.   You've probably heard of the Rorschach test.

Pt.   Yes, I have.

Dr.   I'd like to know what you see. This is the first card.

Pt.   Butterflies.

Dr.   Anything else you see?

Pt.   That's about all.

Dr.   This is the second card.

Pt.   Two animal figures, nothing else.

Dr.   Do you have any ideas about them?

Pt.   No, not really.

Dr.   Perhaps if you turned them upside down you might see something else.

Pt.   (*Long pause.*) No, I'm afraid not.

Dr.   This is the third card.

Pt.   There seem to be two animal figures. That's all.

Dr.   That's the fourth one.

Pt.   Something in the insect family. (*Pause*)

Dr.   This is the fifth card.

Pt.   Represents a sea gull.

Dr.   What makes it a sea gull?

Pt.   The shape.

Dr.   This is the sixth one.

Pt.   I notice one characteristic of all of them, though. You do want me to state what I think?

Dr.   Yes.

Pt.   It's the fact of the similarity to the biological diagrams of a woman's vagina.

Dr.   For instance, where?

Pt.   Right along the edge.

Dr.   Do you see that in any of the others?

Pt.   Yes, I noticed a characteristic in most of them.

Dr.   I see, but you didn't mention that.

Pt.   No.

Dr.   What else do you see?

Pt.   Nothing.

Dr.   This is the seventh.

Pt.   Represents a statue or something. (*Pause*) Looks like two animals perched on top of something or other, that's about all I can get out of it.

Dr.   You see anything else there?

Pt.   No.

Dr. This is the eighth.

Pt. Two lions standing.

Dr. This is the ninth.

Pt. (*Long pause.*) I can't see anything (*Hands card back.*)

Dr. All right, this is the tenth one.

Pt. Squirrels feeding. Tree branches here, and that's all I can get out of it.

Dr. All right, fine. Now I'm going to come back and ask you a few questions. In this one, (*second card*) you saw two animals there. What are the animals doing?

Pt. They're holding up their paws.

Dr. Do the red spots have any significance?

Pt. No.

Dr. How about this?

Pt. Ah, a butterfly.

Dr. Where would you say the female genitals were?

Pt. Well, they're covered.

Dr. Where?

Pt. That's the way they're turned in like.

Dr. Would the thigh be somewheres?

Pt. Yes, right along here.

Dr. What could this red part be?

Pt. It could be blood from an intercourse.

Dr. Blood from an intercourse? I'm going to show you the next card, that's the third one. You mentioned there were two animals, what are they doing?

Pt. Well it's just like a pose.

Dr. Just like a pose. Now what about the red spots there, what could those be?

Pt. Well I couldn't say.

Dr. I'm going to show you this card, the ninth card that you couldn't see anything in. Now look closely and tell me the first thought that comes to you.

Pt. Well that too, might be the walls of the woman's vagina.

Dr. Anything else?

Pt. No.

Dr. Now I'm going to give you a paper and I'd like to have you draw me a picture of a person.

Pt. I don't suppose I'm very good at drawing.

Dr. I see you've got the head of a man there. Supposing you draw me the picture of a woman. (*Patient draws a crude picture of a woman's head.*)

(*It is quite apparent from the tests that the patient is severely neurotic, that he has problems in relationships with people, that he conceives of intercourse as a bloody act. He masters his anxiety by minimizing his productivity, by detachment, and by an intellectual attitude toward life. Self-esteem is markedly inhibited and assertiveness very low. One defense that the patient has is avoiding the fact that he has any real problems. It would obviously be futile to do any therapeutic work on his basic problems until he becomes aware of them and is motivated to correct them. His present motivation is to eliminate his sexual defect, and he does not wish to go any deeper.*)

Dr. From your history, from the way things have been going with you, you feel everything has been perfectly normal except this one symptom, premature ejaculation. You would be happy to have everything remain at its present level if your sexual relations could be better?

Pt. Yes.

Dr. There is no other problem that you would want corrected?

Pt. No.

Dr. There seem to be some indications from the Rorschach that there are other problems that involve your relationships with people. For instance, there are indications that you detach yourself a little bit more than is good for you, in the attempt to avoid stimulating situations. Almost as if in keeping apart from them nothing bad will happen. Of course, these tests could be wrong, they are merely indications.

Pt. I see.

Dr. There are indications also of an overevaluation of the intellectual aspects of life to a minimization of the more emotional aspects.

Pt. Yes.

Dr. This could include the sexual element too. Now what we have to decide on is what our objective will be in treatment. Are we just going to shoot at the sexual symptom, or are we going to shoot at the broader issue of your relationships with people, which would be a much more ambitious procedure, and involve a much longer period of time?

Pt.   Well that's the difficulty, doctor. You see, I don't have much time to devote now. And I'm in a terrible state right now as far as time is concerned to have this thing checked before it goes too long. That's what I'm up against.

Dr.   What do you mean time?

Pt.   Well for one thing, it's hard getting away from my business, of course, and then evenings it would be difficult to get away.

Dr.   I see.

Pt.   And I want to get over this before it gets worse. Of course the period of time enters into it, something I should have done a long time ago I mean; instead I waited.

Dr.   Well I can tell you that there are other problems that you have besides sexual ones, but that if you'd like to work hypnotically with only the sexual thing we can do so.

Pt.   Yes.

Dr.   Tackle this one thing and leave the others alone.

Pt.   Yes, I think for the time being at any rate.

Dr.   Always with the idea that I may be able to present you with more data about what I think about yourself, the significance of which you can evaluate.

Pt.   Yes.

Dr.   I think we will need a period of ten sessions to see if we are going to be successful, or if other things have to be worked through before we can be successful. In other words, if it's not bound up with other problems it will be corrected. But if it's intermeshed with many other problems which involve your relationships with people, it may take a longer time.

Second Session (April 2)

In this session the patient brings up masturbatory misconceptions. These are clarified and an attempt made to correct them. The ideas about masturbation are presented in an authoritarian manner since the motivations of the patient will allow of no other approach at this time. Hypnosis is induced and a medium trance

achieved. The patient appears to be quite responsive to sugges-
tions. The nature of his hypnotically induced dreams indicates
what the Rorschach brought out: passivity and impaired biologic
drives.

Dr.　Have you been thinking about our last talk?

Pt.　Yes.

Dr.　Did you have any other ideas after I had talked to you?

Pt.　No.

Dr.　Or any thoughts?

Pt.　I thought that masturbation could have been the cause.

Dr.　Could you tell me something about your masturbation,
when it started, what fantasies were associated with it and so forth.

Pt.　Well, it started in early childhood, about ten or eleven years.
I might have been about ten or twelve.

Dr.　Do you remember the circumstances under which it started?

Pt.　No, no.

Dr.　And what happened?

Pt.　Well it was just the imagination of, oh, sexual intercourse.

Dr.　Do you still have sexual intercourse fantasies with masturbation?

Pt.　That's right.

Dr.　Any erection trouble with masturbation?

Pt.　No.

Dr.　Any fears associated with it?

Pt.　No.

Dr.　Do you have any conscious fears about sexual intercourse?

Pt.　No.

Dr.　Any thoughts or fantasies occur when you want to engage in
intercourse?

Pt.　No. Well, the same as any other men feel, the desire is there,
it's frequent.

Dr.　Is there a desire to penetrate?

Pt.　That's right.

Dr.　I see. Now why do you think that masturbation was the
cause?

Pt.　Well years back, I mean, in earliest periodicals and literature, I found things that hinted at masturbation being the cause

of physical harm. At that time and in earlier youth I felt as though there's nothing that could be done about it. It was only later on after I read further and found that there could be, that something could be done about it. That's when I started investigating.

Dr. In other words, you had read material to the effect that masturbation can cause premature ejaculation?

Pt. That's right. Of course maybe I was under the impression that it was the, the fundamental cause of impotency in man. That's why I feared and shied away from any serious thought of marriage.

Dr. I see.

Pt. Until one day when I read otherwise.

Dr. How about the frequency of masturbation?

Pt. Well, that's hard to say.

Dr. How frequently did you used to masturbate when you were a boy?

Pt. As often, I should say, at the rate of about three times a week.

Dr. Three times a week, and that continued through when?

Pt. Yes, it's continued through to a later period in the twenties.

Dr. How about now?

Pt. No.

Dr. When did you stop masturbating?

Pt. About five years ago.

Dr. Do you think that masturbation is a normal or abnormal thing?

Pt. I've always considered it abnormal until I consulted this physician who told me that there was nothing abnormal about it.

Dr. Did that surprise you?

Pt. Yes, it did. It did.

Dr. Did you know that practically all children masturbate? Boys and girls?

Pt. No, I didn't know that; it's only at a recent date that I discovered that a good percentage of them do. I always thought it was the exception.

Dr. Masturbation is the yielding to the sexual impulse that is normally present in all children. Almost universally children are led to feel that it is evil.

Pt. That's right.

Dr. It is extremely important that your misconceptions about masturbation be clarified and corrected. We will have the best chance to overcome your symptom when we do this.

Pt. I see. I might add this, which might be helpful. As I say, all through the periods of years I felt that due to a long period of masturbation I thought that the difficulty was purely organic and that it could not be cured, and I was so amazed when I found that it was nothing organic at all, that it was something that was built up in the mind. Especially in my particular case and that it might have caused a barrier.

Dr. The effects of this misconception probably did. But even though we correct the misconceptions, it may take time for you to overcome years of fear. Not long ago there was a tradition of guilt about sex so profound that all text books and all literature decried the evils of masturbation. There were times when books were written to that effect which were completely fantastic, utterly opposed to science, utterly opposed to biology, and utterly opposed to facts.

Pt. I see.

Dr. Now, I am going to give you certain scientific facts for what they may be worth on masturbation. But whether you utilize them and whether they can immediately disperse your old misconceptions is an entirely different story. A child, when he's very little, is entirely dependent upon the parents. When he's little he has no other way of life. In the course of his development and growth, the normal child eventually will give up much of his dependency and become independent and assertive. He does this by exploring his environment and finding pleasures within himself, and his own capacities to do things through his own efforts rather than to get things from the parent. That's part of the normal growth of the individual.

Pt. Yes.

Dr. Now, what occurs is that as his brain develops, the child becomes more and more cognizant of his own body. He gradually explores himself, his feet, his eyes, and even his genitals which are, after all, part of him.

Pt. Yes.

Dr.   The genitals are very delicate and sensitive.

Pt.   Sensitive.

Dr.   And he gets a certain pleasure sensation from the handling that is perfectly normal. Biologically it is important because it serves to teach the child that he can find pleasures within himself, that he doesn't need all pleasures from the parent. So that it serves as one way of beginning to break his dependency on the parent, the mother in particular, for all kinds of gratifications. In the course of genital manipulation, the child finds that the pleasures he gets serve as a means of alleviating tension.

Pt.   That's right.

Dr.   That adds to the growth of the self, ego growth we call it. It's perfectly normal. Mind you the child does not make a career out of masturbating. He merely manipulates his genitals occasionally; at first out of curiosity, then for pleasure. When he finds other pleasure outlets, genital manipulation does not become too important. But if the parent restrains the child, if the parent punishes the child—which many sexually repressed parents do—it teaches the child that there's something evil and bad, not only about his sex organs, but more importantly about doing things for himself and finding pleasures within himself and through his own resources. He is apt then to feel that being independent is bad or dangerous, and he may cling to his dependency strivings.

Pt.   I see.

Dr.   Now, as the child develops, the sexual feeling continues to be strong. Tension builds up. This is particularly the case during puberty when the sex organs mature. Masturbation is the usual outlet for these tensions due to the fact that sexual intercourse is, for social and economic reasons, taboo. Where the child has no great guilt feelings about masturbation, he will relieve his tension without fear. Where such guilt feelings exist, tension may drive him to masturbation, but the aftermath is disastrous. He hates himself and his parents and the world. He believes himself doomed to eternal suffering, and feels that he has, through masturbation, injured himself physically.

Pt.   What you say, doctor, I know is right, because when I have been tense I have had the urge.

Dr.   The release of tension through masturbation, if not ham-

pered becomes no problem at all. But if the child feels restricted
and evil for this impulse, masturbation and sex become a problem. They are overvalued. The greater the restriction, the more
important sex becomes for him, and the more evil he feels.

Pt.   Right.

Dr.   Sex and masturbation may dominate his thinking.

Pt.   That's right.

Dr.   The same could be said for any frustrated biologic drive.
If a hungry person satisfies his appetite, he doesn't think
much about his stomach. But if he is unable to satisfy his appetite, if he remains hungry, his thoughts will be constantly
on food.

Pt.   The child feels it's wrong and bad to masturbate, but he
does anyway.

Dr.   Most authorities feel that the only hurt that can come
through masturbation are the thoughts of evil that are associated with it.

Pt.   Exactly. Well, I did feel all the way through childhood, I
had a terrible sense of guilt and perhaps that's what was built
up in me.

Dr.   It was built up, and nurtured, and gradually gave rise to
many misconceptions about your sex organs.

Pt.   That I do remember vividly, having that terrific sense of
guilt and shame for myself, I mean, all the way through.

Dr.   This guilt and shame reflects itself in other ways. The
Rorschach cards I showed you last time indicate that there is an
association, perhaps unconscious, between sexual intercourse,
blood, and hurt of some kind. There may be misconceptions about
the female sex organs too. There's a link somewhere, and through
hypnosis we may be able to get the answer, to correct that misconception, too. Once we correct the misconceptions of masturbation, sexual relations, and misconceptions in reference to a
woman's sexual organs, you will have the best chance to enter
into a normal sexual relationship. But sometimes it takes a little
time to break a habit.

Pt.   I expect so.

Dr.   But once we have the road cleared we should make progress.

Pt.   I hope so.

Dr. Now I want to talk about hypnosis. Have you ever been hypnotized?

Pt. No, I haven't, but students in the classroom, I've seen it, students being hypnotized.

Dr. I see, you've seen hypnotic process.

Pt. Yes.

Dr. What do you think about hypnosis?

Pt. Well, I, from what I've seen of it and studied of it, I think it's a very valuable science.

Dr. Hypnosis is suggestion.

Pt. That's right.

Dr. And the ability to incorporate suggestion. Practically all people can be hypnotized. It's a matter of concentration.

Pt. Yes.

Dr. Supposing I give you an example of what the hypnotic process is all about. I'd like to have you clasp your hands this way, keep your feet down. Clasp your hands and then, for a moment, close your eyes and imagine that you are looking at a vise. One of those heavy metal vises with jaws that clamp together with a screw. Imagine that your hands are like the jaws of a vise, and that they gradually begin to press together, harder and harder and harder. I'm going to start counting from one to five. When I reach the count of five, your hands will be pressed together so firmly that it will be difficult or impossible to open them up. It will be just like the jaws of that vise. Imagine that you're looking at the vise now, and I begin to count. One, tight; two, tighter; tighter; three, tighter and tighter still; four, as tight as a vise; five, so tight, so firm that they get cemented together. You notice that even when you try to separate them, they're so firmly clasped together that the harder you try, the more firmly they're clasped. And even though you try to pull them apart, they become very closely clasped together, just like that. Now, slowly, they begin to open up, and then you'll be able to open them up. Slowly, they open up. And now you're able to separate them slowly, just like that. Good. Now pull them apart. That is one of the phenomena of hypnosis, the ability to visualize something and feel it is so.

Now another phenomenon is this. Supposing you bring the

palms of your hands down on your thighs and you watch your hands. Watch either hand, say the right hand. I want you to begin experiencing all the sensations and feelings in your hand no matter what they may be. Perhaps you'll feel the sensation of roughness of the trousers on your hand. Perhaps you'll experience sensations; perhaps you'll get little tingling sensations in your fingers. No matter what sensation you feel, I want you to concentrate more and more and more on the feelings in your hands. Just watch your hands.

Now you'll begin to notice an interesting thing. As you watch your hand, you'll notice that one of the fingers will move. You don't know which one of the fingers will move first, whether it will be on the right hand or the left hand. But one of the fingers will move ever so little. It may be the middle finger or the thumb, or the little finger, or the ring finger. Whichever finger it is, it will move soon. You don't know exactly when. It will move and jerk as you watch it. Perhaps you'll notice that the space between the fingers will gradually widen, the fingers spreading apart, the space becoming wider and wider, just like that. And as you notice the space increasing, you'll become aware of the feeling of lightness in your fingers. Your hand and fingers will begin to feel light.

Slowly your hand will begin to lift and rise, slowly rise and lift, lift, pulling up, up higher, and higher so that the hand and fingers lift and rise, slowly rise, up in the air as if they're like a feather. Rising and lifting just like that. Higher and higher and higher; slowly, imperceptibly and even perhaps without your knowledge, the hand will lift up toward your face. It will begin to rise, and you'll begin to feel the sensation of heaviness and sleepiness in your whole body except the right hand.

You'll begin to feel tired, very tired. You'll begin to get drowsy. Your eyes will get heavy, very heavy. They'll get so heavy and tired and sleepy they blink. They blink and you get tired and drowsy.

Your breathing now becomes deeper. The hand continues to rise up, and your breathing gets deep, and your eyes get heavy, and your body gets heavy, and you get sleepier, and sleepier, and sleepier. And as the hand rises, you'll notice that you'll get sleepier all over until when the hand touches your face, you'll be asleep, firmly asleep, deeply asleep. And you'll get drowsier and drowsier and drowsier, and finally when the hand touches your face, lean the cheek against the palm of your hand to support the head and go to sleep, go to sleep. You are tired, very drowsy. Your eyes are blinking. Now your breathing gets deep and automatic. Slowly your hand begins to lift up, up, up, higher, higher, lifting straight to your face, and as it lifts your eyes get so heavy that it's difficult to keep them open. You'll be going into a deep restful sleep. Your hand is moving towards your face, and you're getting drowsier and drowsier and drowsier. You're going to sleep; you're going to sleep; you're going to get sleepier, and sleepier, just like that.

I want you to rest this way for a few minutes, and at the end of that time I'm going to talk to you again, and you're going to be asleep, deeply asleep. And when I talk to you next you'll be much more deeply asleep than you were before. (*Pause*)

As you sit there, I want you to continue to feel the sensation of deep restful sleep. This time I'm going to ask you to open your eyes when I count five and look at a shiny object. When I show it to you, you're going to notice that as you gaze at it, it will be impossible to keep your eyes open, and that the harder you stare at it, the more tired your eyes will get. And finally they'll get so tired that they'll close and again you'll go to sleep, deeply asleep. One, two, three, four, five. Slowly open your eyes and stare at the object, and as you stare at it, your eyes will get heavy. They blink, they burn, they feel like lead, and then, when they feel so tired that it's impossible to keep them open, they'll close and you'll go into a deep restful, relaxed comfortable sleep. Your eyes get tired, they're tired and you get drowsier and drowsier and drowsier. Stare at the object as long as you possibly can. And then your eyes will begin to close and you'll go to sleep. Very tired, tired and drowsy. Get sleepier, very sleepy. Go to sleep, go to sleep, go to sleep. And as you sleep, your whole body will relax, from your head right down to your feet. I want you to sit this way in a deep sleep, drowsy sleep, until I talk to you next. When I talk to you next, you'll be still more asleep than you were before, and I'll give you more suggestions that you'll find it easy to follow. Go to sleep and I'll talk to you soon. (*Pause*)

Now, I'm going to ask you slowly to wake up, and after you

wake up, I'm going to count from one to five. As I count from one to five, at the count of five, you'll notice that your eyes will again have become so heavy that it will be difficult or impossible to keep them open. Slowly open your eyes, and then I'll count. One, they blink, two, they get heavy; three, get drowsy; four, get sleepier and sleepier. They start closing. You get tired. Five, they close. Your breathing gets deep, very deep and automatic.

Now I'm going to start stroking your left hand. You'll notice something very interesting; the left hand will start getting extremely heavy, very heavy, as I stroke it. It will get heavier and heavier and heavier so that it will feel as if a hundred pound weight is pressing down on the arm. It will feel as if two bands strap your arm down, at your elbow and at your wrist. It will feel as if a suction pad pulls your arm down against your body. It will feel as if it's made of lead, heavy and stiff, so that when I reach the count of five, it will feel so heavy that even when I try to budge it, it will feel heavy and stiff, and it will be impossible for you to lift it. It will be impossible for you to lift it. I may, by pulling it, possibly get it up a little bit. It will come down, but it won't lift up. One, heavy; two, heavier and heavier; three, as heavy as lead. Visualize a heavy stiff lead bar. Four, heavier and heavier; five, heavy and stiff. The muscles become rigid and stiff so that when I try to pull it up, it stiffens up just like that. And the harder I pull, the stiffer it gets. You'll notice now that even though you try to move it, the harder you try to move your arm, the heavier it will feel. The harder you try to move your arm, the heavier it will feel.

I'm going, now, to count from one to five. At the count of five, you'll find that you are able to move your arm. It will lose its stiffness, and you will be able to move it. One, two, three, four, five. Good. And now you're going to notice an extremely interesting thing. You're going to notice that as you sit there, you'll feel your arm so heavy and stiff that it will be impossible for you to move it. But this time you, yourself, will count from one to five, and when you reach the count of five, you'll notice that suddenly the arm will loosen up and get limp and you will be able to move it. At the same time your eyes will continue to be closed, and you go into an even deeper state of sleep. So count from one to five.

At the count of five, you notice suddenly the arm will be able to move.

(The purpose of this technic is to start giving the patient a feeling of capacity of controlling muscular function as a means of building up a feeling of self-confidence, to show him he is not entirely helpless about influencing his physical self.)

Pt. One, two, three, four, five.

Dr. You can move your arm now, good. Now I want you to go to sleep even deeper, and in a few minutes, I'm going to talk to you again. *(Pause)* Now, as you sit there, I'm going to give you a suggestion. Visualize yourself walking along a street with me. We go along together, we walk toward a churchyard. We enter the churchyard. We notice a tall church in front of us, the spire and steeple. As you visualize that, indicate the fact that you see it by your hand rising up about two inches. As soon as you visualize ourselves walking along the street to the churchyard, indicate it by your hand rising up. Your hand rises up.

As you observe the church, the spire and the steeple, notice a bell. The bell begins to move. You get a sensation as if you hear the bell clanging. As soon as you get that sensation indicate it by your hand rising up. Your hand rises up.

Now I'm going to ask you to wake up slowly, as I count from one to five. At the count of five, you still will be drowsy, but your eyes will be awake, open. And then, after that, I'm going to say "Sleep, sleep, sleep, sleep," and as I say "Sleep," your eyes again will become very heavy and tired, so heavy that it will be impossible to keep them open. And then they'll close very tightly. One, slowly start opening your eyes; two; three; four; five. Sleep, sleep, sleep, sleep; your eyes are tired and heavy, and you're going into a deeper and deeper and more restful, more relaxed, more comfortable sleep.

As you sit there this time, you'll notice that your entire body becomes heavy, heavy, very heavy and stiff; it's almost as if it's frozen. I'm going to count from one to five; at the count of five, your body will be so heavy and stiff and cramped that when you try to get out of the chair, it will be impossible for you to move out of the chair no matter how hard you try. It will be impossible for you to get out of the chair. One, heavy; two, stiff; three, heavier and heavier; four, as heavy as lead, as heavy as lead, as heavy as lead; five, it's heavy and stiff. No matter how hard you try to move or to budge or to wiggle in your chair, the harder you try the more solidly implanted you are in your chair. Try it and you'll see that the harder you try the more stiff you get. Your whole body begins to stiffen up.

And now, I'm going to ask you again to count from one to five. As you, yourself, count from one to five, at the count of five, even though you're deeply asleep, it will be possible for you to move a little in the chair. Count.

Pt.   One, two, three, four, five.

Dr.   You can move, good. Now I'm going to ask you to visualize something again. This time I approach you and I have a bottle in my hand. You notice that there is a label on the bottle with a flower printed on it. Imagine that there is perfume in the bottle. As soon as you visualize the bottle and label and flower, indicate it by your hand rising. Your hand rises. Now I'm going to unscrew the cork on the bottle and bring it close to your nose. You'll actually be able to smell the odor of perfume. As soon as you do indicate it by your hand moving up. Your hand rises.

Imagine now that you are in a surgeon's office, because of a finger that has become very, very painful. Your finger has a boil on it, and the doctor says it's necessary to open it. It's necessary to make an incision in the finger, in order to relieve the pressure, in order to take out the pus. And, in order to do that, he injects novocaine around the wrist, like this, to create a wrist block, anesthesia of the hand. So the feeling in the hand will get numb. There will be no feeling of pain.

As you sit there, imagine that your hand has been injected and that you feel as if you're wearing a thick, heavy leather glove. I'm going to count from one to five, and as I reach the count of five, you'll notice that you get a sensation of wearing a thick heavy leather glove. The feeling will be so real that it will be as if you're actually wearing a thick heavy leather glove. As I count to five, you get the sensation that your hand is different from the other hand, that it's wearing a glove. As soon as you get the impression or feeling that your hand is wearing a thick, heavy leather glove, indicate it by your hand rising up in the air—like that.

You'll notice that whereas the right hand is sensitive, this hand begins to feel numb even when I prick it deeply. (*The hand is pricked with a needle.*) You notice that? Even when I prick it deeply there's a numbness here. Any pain?

Pt. No.

Dr. As you sit there, I'm going to suggest to you that you imagine yourself in a theater observing a play. You're sitting in the audience, and you notice the stage in front of you. The curtain is drawn. Now I'm going to count from one to five, and at the count of five suddenly the curtains will be drawn apart, and you'll see action on the stage. You'll visualize a play. No matter what you visualize, tell me about it without waking up. As soon as I reach the count of five, you'll see a flash of action. One, two, three, four, five.

Pt. It's in a green sitting room.

Dr. Yes?

Pt. Somebody's sitting at the piano, playing.

Dr. What?

Pt. Two other people reading.

(*As in his response to the Rorschach cards, movement in this fantasy is minimal. A restriction of creativeness, activity and biologic drive is suggested.*)

Dr. A scene, a quiet living room scene. What you have visualized is a fantasy. Fantasies and dreams are of the same caliber, except dreams are more vivid, but they're essentially the same. Now tonight when you go to sleep you'll notice that you probably will dream. You probably will dream, and if you do remember the dream, I want you to bring it in to me. Tonight when you go to bed you will dream, and if you do remember the dream, bring it in with you when you come to see me next.

Now, next time we try this I'm going to repeat "Sleep, sleep, sleep, sleep," and as I do, you'll notice that your eyes will get heavier and heavier and heavier, and finally they'll close, and you'll go into a sleep which will get progressively deeper and deeper.

As you sit there, now, I'm going to give you the suggestion that you have a dream or an image that is like a dream. As soon as you've had that, indicate it by your hand rising, lifting. As soon as you've had a dream or fantasy that's like a dream, indicate it by your hand rising, no matter how long it takes. *(Pause)* Now your hand rises.

Listen carefully to me. When you wake up, you may or may not remember the fantasy or dream that you've had. It makes no difference. If you remember it, tell it to me. You may not remember other things that happened; it's immaterial. But this is important, when you wake up, you'll notice that when you look at me, your eyes will begin blinking, that it will be impossible to look at me without your eyes jerking and blinking. I'm going to count from one to five, and when I reach the count of five, your eyes will open up, and you'll blink. No matter how hard you try to control it, the spasms will continue. You'll not be able to stop yourself from blinking. Then I'm going to say, "Close your eyes," following which I'll say, "Slowly open them." And this time your eyes will not blink when you look at me. This time you'll notice that your eyes will not blink when you look at me. The first time they will, and then I'll ask you to close them, and the second time they will not blink. One; at the count of five open your eyes. They will blink spastically as you look at me; two, three, four, five. Notice how your eyes are blinking? Now close them. Slowly, as you open them now, it will be possible for you to look at me without your eyes blinking. Good. Good. How do you feel?

Pt.   Sleepy.

Dr.   Fine, what do you remember?

Pt.   Meeting my wife, taking her out walking to the theater, a dream.

Dr.   Fine, now tomorrow we meet again at four-fifteen.

Pt.   Four-fifteen.

THIRD SESSION (APRIL 3)

Patient has a dream, in response to my suggestion, which indicates he is putting me in a paternal role. In hypnosis an attempt is made to analyze what may be behind his lack of penial sensations in intercourse. He exhibits resistance to this probing, and obviously does not wish to analyze. Suggestive and persuasive commands are given him to adopt a different attitude toward sexual relations.

Pt. It is amazing. I did have somewhat of a dream last night. I don't really remember it well. It is very short, too vague. It is a peculiar thing, I dreamt of my father, and it is the first time I have. It didn't consist of very much.

Dr. Can you tell me what it was?

Pt. Yes. I was walking into a church, and he was sitting there and sort of made room for me to sit next to him. I don't remember very much—there wasn't very much beyond that.

Dr. I see.

Pt. But I saw him sitting there, and naturally I walked over to sit down along side of him.

Dr. Do you have any association to walking into church?

Pt. Well, I have been going to church more. In my youth I did attend services with my Dad. He was religious and I always managed to attend with him.

Dr. And with your Dad do you recall a certain feeling of closeness?

Pt. Closeness? Yes.

Dr. Now, did your Dad demand that you go to church?

Pt. No, he didn't have to. I mean I knew that he desired it that way and I went. And I rather liked it—I mean—it was nice—the associations with home.

Dr. You were quite fond of your Dad?

Pt. Yes.

Dr. Your fantasies about your Dad, are they always of a pleasant variety?

Pt. Yes. Very.

Dr. Did you have any other feelings or ideas in relation to him?

Pt. No. After I left you I thought of him.

(In response to my suggestion the patient had a dream which turns out to be a transference dream. Apparently the patient desires and expects me to play a paternal role. If his feelings

toward his father are not too ambivalent, he may be very respon-
sive to prestige suggestion.)

Dr. What happened when you left?

Pt. I went home. I didn't tell my wife I came to see you. We tried sex.

Dr. What happened?

Pt. Well, the same thing.

Dr. Can you describe that more in detail?

Pt. Well, yes. After about 10 or 15 minutes of preliminaries I tried to insert it.

Dr. You had an erection?

Pt. That's right. And upon insertion it was the same thing—I—it lasted for I should say a little over a half minute—between a half minute and a minute.

Dr. Between a half minute and a minute. You inserted your penis?

Pt. That's right.

Dr. Did you get any sensation when you inserted it?

Pt. No, no.

Dr. Did you get any feeling of pleasure, or did you get any feeling of pressure; was it anesthetic or what?

Pt. It was almost anesthetic.

Dr. Almost anesthetic.

Pt. Yes. The feeling of pleasure is somewhat, I imagine, secondary, because of the tension that I'm under at that particular moment. You see, that fear is always there with me. Will I succeed or will I not succeed?

Dr. The fear that you will or will not succeed is there.

Pt. Fear that I won't succeed.

Dr. I see. Then the insertion isn't so much the desire for pleasure as it is wondering about the success.

Pt. That's right. That is the thing.

Dr. So that you never have actually permitted yourself to feel any sensations in intercourse.

Pt. That's right. That's exactly what it is.

Dr. Now yesterday, briefly, before we started hypnosis, we emphasized several things. First, the masturbatory misconceptions, and, second, the fact that there may be other elements operating of which you may not be aware. Now we're not going to work in too great detail because you don't want to change everything. We want to accomplish as much as we can in as little time as possible. I'm going to give you strong suggestions that will enable you to function sexually. If your difficulty is not too deep, these will enable you to function. If it is on a more complicated basis, it may be necessary to go into more material.

Pt. I see.

Dr. One thing that may be essential is to capture fantasies or associations that occur in the process of inserting your penis.

Pt. Yes.

Dr. We may possibly do that under hypnosis. What I'm going to have you do is work out a plan, an ordered plan of establishing a better contact with your wife in order that you overcome whatever fears there may be.

Pt. Yes.

Dr. Has she read any medical books on sex?

Pt. Yes, she has.

Dr. How about yourself, have you read anything?

Pt. Some things, not much.

Dr. I'm going to give you a list of books. Perhaps you and your wife can read to remove as many misconceptions as possible about the sexual function and the sexual act.

Pt. I see.

Dr. Now, we will use hypnosis again. Did you feel relaxed yesterday?

Pt. Yes. I was wondering, doctor, is there any way of knowing, am I susceptible to suggestion, or is it just my willingness to cooperate? I mean I have no way of telling.

Dr. Whether you are complying voluntarily or automatically in a trance is not material. It is not necessary for you to comply. Actually every person who is hypnotized asks these questions about hypnosis. It is not necessary that you concern yourself too much with them. The way we're utilizing hypnosis here is not so much in a sense of creating a sense of passivity, a sense of compliance, but rather of you participating with me to achieve certain effects

and a certain mastery of functions. As you proceed you will get
the idea.

Pt. Yes.

Dr. It will be possible for you to control your own functions
and, through the medium of hypnosis, you, yourself, will begin
to be able to master certain sensations and functions. You will be
able to translate that over into the sexual area, eventually.

Pt. I see.

Dr. All right, now supposing you lean back in your chair and
again bring your hands down and watch your fingers; watch your
fingers, and as you watch your fingers, this time rapidly, you'll
begin to notice that your hand will get light, that the fingers will
slowly lift up in the air, and that you will begin to sleep, sleep,
sleep, sleep. Your eyes will get heavy and then close and your
hand will lift up toward your face, straight up. Just like that.
And when it touches your face, lean your head up against the palm
of your hand and go to sleep. It is moving up, you are getting
drowsier and drowsier and drowsier. Sleep, sleep, sleep, sleep,
sleep. You're very tired. Very tired. Drowsy, drowsy, very drowsy.
From your head right down to your feet. You're going to get so
tired and drowsy and sleepy. You are going into a deep restful
sleep. Your hand is moving up, up, up, straight up to your face.
Your whole body is heavy except for your arm. You get drowsier
and drowsier and drowsier. As soon as your hand touches your
face, just relax and sleep. Now you are asleep. Sleep for a few
minutes and then I'll talk to you again. You'll be more deeply
asleep. *(Pause)*

As you sit there, I'm going to stroke your arm, your other arm,
and as I do you'll begin to notice that it gets heavy, very heavy,
and that the heaviness sweeps down, right down, from your
shoulder to your finger tips, so that the arm gets just as heavy
as lead and stiff, stiff, just like a board. Heavy and stiff. Heavy and
stiff. As I stroke it, it gets heavier and heavier and heavier. I'm
going to count from one to five, and at the count of five, it will
feel so stiff and rigid that even when I try to budge it, it will not
move. One, heavy; two, heavier and heavier; three, as heavy and
stiff as a board; four, stiffer and stiffer and heavier; five, just as

heavy as a board. When I try to budge it, it remains heavy and stiff, and you yourself will notice that even though you try to budge it, the harder you try, the heavier it will feel, until the muscles become so achy and so heavy that it is impossible to lift it.

At the same time, your entire body begins to feel heavy and stiff and rigid, almost as if you're made of iron. I'm going to count from one to five, and at the count of five, you'll notice that your entire body will have become so heavy and so stiff that even though you try to budge out of the chair, you cannot. You'll notice that the harder you try the heavier you feel. One, heavy; two, stiff; three, heavier and heavier; four, as heavy as lead; five, heavy and stiff, and when you try to move out of your chair, the harder you try, the heavier and stiffer you get, so that it is impossible to budge even though you try. It is impossible to budge. Try and you'll see that the harder you try to get up, the heavier you feel.

Now as you sit there, I'm going to ask you, yourself, to count from one to five, and you'll notice that now that you count from one to five, at the count of four it will be impossible for you to move your body or arm, but at the count of five, your body will relax, so that it will be possible for you to move your body and to move your arm. Go ahead.

Pt.   One, two, three, four . . . five.

Dr.   Now you can move your arm and body. You noticed that, didn't you?

Pt.   Yes.

Dr.   Good. Now I'm going to ask you, as you sit there, to visualize yourself again walking with me toward the church, and as we walk you go into the churchyard, you see the tall spires and steeples and the bell. As soon as you hear the ringing of the bell, your hand will rise to indicate that to me. (*Hand rises.*) Now it comes down again, and you begin to feel more tired and more sleepy, drowsier and drowsier and drowsier.

In a moment I'm going to count from one to five, and at the count of five, this time, your eyes will open up, but you will still feel drowsy. You'll still feel sleepy, and the moment I say, "Sleep, sleep, sleep," your eyelids will feel just like lead, and even though you try to keep them open, you'll notice that your eyes shut firmly. One, two, three, four, five—sleep, sleep, sleep—your eyes shut.

Now listen carefully to me. I'm going to stroke your hand again, and I want you to go to sleep and to dream. It may take a little time or it may come shortly. You'll have a dream, and this time your dream will indicate your feelings, your deep feelings about your father, no matter what they may be. The dream will be about your deep feelings about your father. As soon as you have that dream, your hand will rise to indicate that to me. Continue to sleep, continue to sleep, continue to sleep. I want you to sleep. Perhaps you'll visualize the scene on the stage, by looking at the stage and noticing the curtain opening up. I want you to report to me exactly what you see. No matter what it is that you see. It will appear just like a dream, because a dream is nothing more than thoughts that occur in a state of sleep. I want you to tell me about it as soon as you see that, indicating that you've seen it by your hand rising. (*Hand rises.*) Like that. Go ahead now. I want you to tell me just what you dreamed. What did you see?

Pt.   Father sitting on a chair, reading the paper. People sitting around the table playing cards.

(*The passive content of the dream will be noted.*)

Dr.   Good. Now as you sit there, I'm going to give you some suggestions. It is essential for you at this point to begin to have certain feelings restored to you. You have a desire to function, to function well sexually. Your left hand will move, will rise about two inches, if you have that desire. It will be able to rise if you have the desire to function well sexually. (*Hand rises.*) You have that desire, your hand moves and now you bring it down.

If you have the desire to function sexually as you indicate, then it will be possible to remove the causes that prevent you from functioning sexually. It will be possible to do that in two ways; understanding what is blocking you from functioning sexually, and retraining yourself, so that you can function well sexually. Now if you have a real desire to overcome this, and I believe you have—you've indicated it to me—then you will have the desire to go into whatever feelings and whatever fantasies are important. You'll have a desire to tackle this thing.

I want you to visualize yourself in this theater, watching your-self on the stage. This time you will be performing sexually with your wife. You're on the stage, you play with her, you have an erection, and then you insert your penis. You then suddenly get a flash through your mind, thoughts that come to you in a flash about what goes on underneath the surface—fear, disgust or what-ever it is as you insert your penis. As soon as you see this, indicate it to me by your hand rising. (*Hand rises.*) Your hand rises. Tell me about it.

Pt.   It was just an ordinary flash.

Dr.   What was it?

Pt.   Light.

Dr.   A flash of light. A flash of light. What emotion was there with that flash?

Pt.   None.

(*Patient is so severely repressed that he is unable to acknowledge his deeper feelings. I decide at this point to use a more persuasive than analytic approach.*)

Dr.   None. All right. Now listen to me. If there is no emotion of fear, if there is no emotion of disgust, if there is no emotion of a sort that would inhibit you, then it will be possible for you to put into action what I am going to suggest to you. From now on, I want you, when you go to bed with your wife, to go to bed, not with the idea of performing, not with the fear that you may fail, not with the intense desire and expectation that you are going to succeed, but rather not caring anything about your performance. I want you, instead of feeling you've got to satisfy your wife, merely to insert your penis with the idea of seeing what sensations you can get out of the insertion. It will make no difference whether you have an orgasm immediately, no differ-ence whether you can last any length of time. Merely experience whatever feelings, whatever sensations there may be in your penis. In other words, I'm going to give you a very strong sug-gestion, and that is that it will be possible for you to begin to demonstrate to yourself that you can have feelings. Up to this time you functioned with an anesthetized penis. I want you to begin to have certain feelings in your penis, no matter what they may be. I want you to feel less that you are performing, and more that you have sex for whatever pleasure there is. I would like to have you take your wife into confidence and tell her that you are going to work at this thing, not from a feeling that you've got to perform—because the very challenge of performing may block you and cause you to fail—rather you are going to do it from now on with the idea of feeling what pleasure you can get out of it. On that basis, it will not be a challenge to you. It makes no difference who the man is, if he feels challenged, if he feels that he is going to fail, it will interfere with his performance. And I want you to enter into this new relationship with her with the idea of not caring whether you perform well or whether you do not perform well. Do you understand me?

Pt. Yes.

Dr. You understand me thoroughly and are you desirous of working at this from this point of view?

Pt. Yes.

Dr. You believe you will be able to do this?

Pt. Yes.

Dr. Good. I want you to try to do it and to work at it without the idea of succeeding at all, without the idea of a challenge, but merely with the idea of engaging in an activity that may have pleasure values for you. I'm going to make that a strong suggestion. At the same time I want you to observe yourself, to observe what ideas accompany the sexual act, to observe whether any fear appears, to observe whatever ideas occur so that you can tell me about them. When you go home, it will be possible for you to feel that you are experiencing something important. As you sit there, I'm going to suggest that you will feel a sense of strength developing in you. You will feel more self-confident. You will feel better and stronger, better and stronger.

I want you to be more deeply asleep. Feel yourself dozing off and getting very sleepy. When you wake up, when I wake you up, you'll notice that your left arm is stiff, very stiff, very, very stiff. When I yank on it, it will become stiffer and stiffer and stiffer and more rigid. When you wake up, your arm will become so stiff and rigid, that it will be impossible to budge it. It will be impossible to budge it until I say, "Count." When I say, "Count," you'll count from one to five, and you'll notice that at the count of five, it will then be possible to move your arm. When I wake you up, you will notice that the arm is heavy and stiff, hugs your body and that the harder you try to move it, the heavier it feels. But when I say, "Count," you will count from one to five, and at the count of five, the arm will loosen up and then it will be possible to move it. One—start waking up—two, three, four, five. (*Patient awakens and tries to move his arm unsuccessfully.*) Count.

Pt.   One, two, three, four, five.

Dr.   Now you can move your arm. Good. How do you feel?

Pt.   Relaxed.

Dr.   Good. I'm going to repeat what I said to you because some of this may possibly be obscure now. It is very, very essential to work at this systematically. We are going to try in a very short time, to correct a tendency that you've had all your life. You must enter into sexual relations with your wife on the basis that you're not damaged, that you are functioning all right, that whatever is causing your premature ejaculations are the product of misconceptions and fears that go way back in your life that have no bearing on the situation today. You must look upon sex as a pleasure function, and not think of satisfying your wife for the time being. Your not thinking of her will in the long run be beneficial to her. You must stop regarding sexuality as a means of proving yourself because it cannot do that for anyone. The more a person feels he has to perform in sex, the more he feels he's got to succeed, the quicker he's licked. I'd like to have you, until I see you next, experiment and see what feelings you can develop. Look upon it as a pleasure experience. Don't even think about how long it is going to last. Just see what pleasures you can get out of it. Just experience whatever feelings come up. If you want to take your wife into your confidence, so much the better. If you don't want to, all right.

FOURTH SESSION (APRIL 9)

Patient expresses discouragement. He is reassured and an attempt is made to convince him that there is a connection between his symptom and his attitudes toward women. He refuses to admit this. In hypnosis an attempt is made to condition him

*to a firmer control over his physical functions including the sexual
function. Authoritarian, forceful suggestions are used to get him
to divorce his early misconceptions from his present-day life. His
passivity and fear of aggression are brought up and a hobby is
suggested to permit him to express aggression.*

Dr. Well, how are things?

Pt. Not much good.

Dr. Why not?

Pt. I'm afraid I haven't responded to the suggestions you made.
Somehow I acted the same way I always did.

Dr. After all, a pattern of this type that goes so deep has to be
worked at before a change occurs. It never comes immediately.
Have patience, it will come if you have a strong enough desire.

Pt. I have that.

Dr. You just can't take a lifetime and throw it out the window
in a few days. How long have you been coming here now?

Pt. A little over a week.

Dr. Knowing the path along which to move and not being so
concerned about immediate results is important.

Pt. Yes.

Dr. When did you have relations?

Pt. Last night.

Dr. Well, what thoughts came to you during this? Did you
have any ideas or thoughts about it?

Pt. No, no, there's only one thought at all times that's utmost
in my mind, and it's the eagerness to succeed, to prove, to bring
home to myself that I'm perfectly normal. That was the thought
that was always in my mind. I can't seem to grasp any other
thoughts.

Dr. The thought has been to prove yourself.

Pt. That's right exactly.

Dr. What sort of person is your wife? Can you describe to me
the feelings you have for her, the kind of relationship you have
with her?

Pt. Well, I don't know if I can put it into words very well. I
mean it's a closeness, the intimacy is there naturally, and there's
a great fondness and admiration we have for each other. If I

might add the mere fact that she is so lovely. I'm just, of course—
I know it must mean an awful lot to her. She pretends it doesn't,
and she's perfectly willing to be patient and all that stuff. Which
makes me that much more eager. I mean, had she probably, ah,
well let's see now, how will I put it? Well, had she seemed more
disappointed, more disillusioned, perhaps I would feel differently.
Dr. How would you feel then?
Pt. Well, oh, I feel as though if that's the way it is, I wouldn't
care so much. It would just have to right itself, yes or no, I would
have to gamble on the outcome of it.
Dr. In other words you wouldn't be so eager.
Pt. Eager, exactly. The mere fact that she's so lovely about it,
so fine, so patient.
Dr. Supposing you never succeeded in having relations with her.
What do you fantasy?
Pt. I don't know. At first, well for the first two or three weeks
of our married life, I thought it would end up in an annulment.
You hear about these things and it's logical to assume that your
case will not be different from anybody else's. Of course that was
a terrible thought, and I succeeded in dismissing that mostly, I
think, because in her attitude, I mean, whereby she feels that the
sex angle is that while it's of great importance, it's not of paramount importance. And, she's very much in love with me, and
she admires me and all that sort of thing. Of course, I, as a man,
know the other thing plays a very important part, and marriage
based without that simply can't succeed. Well, I'm not as I was
the first two or three weeks.
Dr. You did talk to her then? And are you convinced that even
though you are never able to have complete relations, she won't
leave you?
Pt. Yes, I really am.
Dr. You're sure?
Pt. So far, yes.
Dr. All right, now we have to go on because you do want to
break this thing up.
Pt. Um hum.
Dr. First, it's good that you feel that she's not going to leave you

under any circumstances. That will prevent you from getting too anxious.

Pt. That's right.

Dr. Second, it will be good for you to feel that you mustn't perform, that there's no challenge. It has nothing to do with your masculinity. It's a problem. You're not impotent, because you do have erections.

Pt. That's right.

Dr. And it's merely the fact that just as soon as you insert, you have an ejaculation.

Pt. That's right.

Dr. We're working on a basis of giving you a certain sense of mastery over your impulses, but at the same time it's necessary to divest you of fears, misconceptions about your own functioning. You are not damaged. Look, if it were true that masturbation produced this in you, then you wouldn't be able to have an erection when you kissed her, hugged her and made love to her.

Pt. I see.

Dr. So that the masturbation thing has nothing to do with this picture. There seems to be a peculiar association to the female genital organ.

Pt. Um hum.

Dr. And the contact with the female genital organ, whatever that happens to mean to you.

Pt. Yes.

Dr. And it may have a content and a meaning to you of a particular kind that is different than for other people.

Pt. I see.

Dr. What about your attitudes towards female sex organs?

Pt. Well, I've never given it much thought. My passion is the same as everybody else's, I suppose.

Dr. By that you mean what?

Pt. The same as any man's thought on these things.

Dr. Well, what do you feel about it? I mean on a conscious level.

Pt. Well, I, I don't know how to put it. What do you mean when you say, how do I feel about it?

Dr. Does it repulse you, do you get frightened by it?

Pt.   No, no.

Dr.   Do you feel excited by it?

Pt.   No.

Dr.   Do you feel it's nasty?

Pt.   No, no, no.

Dr.   You don't have any feelings.

Pt.   No. None.

Dr.   Neither positive nor negative.

Pt.   No, neither positive or negative.

Dr.   Just an indifference?

Pt.   That's right.

Dr.   Behind that indifference there may lie certain fears.

Pt.   Um hum.

Dr.   Because things like this don't happen by magic. The fact that it's disassociated and disconnected from what's going on in your conscious life doesn't mean that it's not there.

Pt.   Yes.

Dr.   Here you have an erection, and just as soon as it comes in contact with the female sex organ it disappears.

Pt.   That's right.

Dr.   Yes, so that it's the contact with the female organ; and what I'm trying to do is to establish a connection and a continuity between the act and the symptom.

Pt.   Um hum.

Dr.   So that if there is any fear, we can bring it up into consciousness and you can get rid of it.

Pt.   That's right.

Dr.   But actually you have, you feel, no associations to the female sex organs that are either repulsive or exciting.

Pt.   I've never felt, not consciously at any rate, I've never felt any repulsion or fear.

Dr.   Well, it may not be there, or it may. And what about your relationships with women in the past? Have you been attracted to any particular type of woman?

Pt.   No.

Dr.   Say a passive type of woman or an active type of woman, what kind of woman has appealed to you?

Pt.   The passive type, more or less.

Dr. And your wife is a passive type?

Pt. That's right.

Dr. Now supposing you just relax yourself and breathe in deeply and then go to sleep. Sleep, sleep, sleep. As you sit there you're going to feel tired and drowsy, and slowly, automatically, even perhaps without your knowledge, your hand, your right hand will lift up. It will rise towards your face, begin to lift and rise, slowly rise and lift as you get sleepier, and sleepier, and sleepier. Very tired and drowsy and sleepy, from your head right down to your feet. Your hand will begin to rise and lift straight up towards your face, and you'll go into a deep restful, relaxed, comfortable sleep. Slowly the hand will rise, and lift. Your eyes get heavy, you get tired and sleepy. The hand is moving up now, moving up, rising straight up towards the face, and when it touches your face, you'll be asleep, in a deep sleep. Very tired, very sleepy. (*Pause*) Now as you sit there, I'm going to ask you to begin counting slowly from one to five. This time, as you count slowly, from one to five, your arm, your left arm, will begin to stiffen up, and to get heavy, so that at the count of five, no matter how hard you try, the arm will have gotten so stiff and so heavy that it will be rigid and will not move. It will not move. It will not relax even though you may try hard to make it relax. It will stay glued up against your thigh. Count slowly, and as you count, your arm will begin to get heavier and heavier and heavier, and it will get so heavy and so stiff that it will not move.

Pt. One, two, three, four, five.

Dr. Notice how heavy and stiff and rigid it is. I'm going to pull at it now, and try to budge it, and it will become stiffer and stiffer and stiffer. And as you sit there, you begin to notice more and more that the arm stiffness continues almost apart from you. Without any participation on your part it continues to be stiff and rigid until you, yourself, give yourself the command to move it by counting from one to five. Now start counting, from one to five, and as you count from one to five, the rigidity will gradually leave. As you count from one to five, the rigidity will gradually leave.

Pt. One, two, three, four, five.

Dr. The arm can move. Now, the arm will stiffen again through your own suggestion. Count from one to five. As you count from one to five, the arm will stiffen and remain in a fixed position, it will stiffen and remain in that position. Even though you try to move it in either direction, it will remain exactly as it is, stiff and rigid and firm. Count from one to five.

Pt.   One, two, three, four, five.

Dr.   You notice how stiff it is? And when you try to budge it, it remains exactly as it is, and it will get stiffer and stiffer and stiffer, and it's impossible for it to go down. It remains stiff, it remains stiff, and it remains rigid just as it is now. And the harder you try to bring it down, the stiffer and heavier it becomes. Now it's possible for you to control that, the stiffness, and the rigidity; it's possible for it to remain stiff and rigid. And you're going to notice this, that it will be possible for you to control all your body functions better and better, even the function of your penis, which too, eventually, will become stiff and rigid when you insert it in the vagina. So that when you insert it in the vagina, you will be able to feel that it remains stiff and rigid, that it continues to be stiff and rigid, just like your arm remains stiff and rigid, and that no matter what happens, it continues to remain stiff and rigid and firm. And I'm going to ask you now to count from one to five, and at the count of five, you will be able to move your arm down to the body.

Pt.   One, two, three, four, five.

Dr.   Now, your arm moves down to your thigh. I want you to sit back in the chair, breathe in deeply and go to sleep deeper. In a few minutes I'll talk to you, and you'll be still more deeply asleep. (*Pause*)

As you sleep, listen to me. Eventually you will liberate yourself from whatever fears, whatever anxieties there exist in your relationship to women, and in your contact with the female sex organs. It makes no difference about the origin of the anxieties. It makes no difference how strong the anxieties are. It will be possible for you to dissociate your own feelings from your fears, if there are fears. Let us assume that there is something that is operating within you, say a childhood misunderstanding or fear of the female sex organs. We do not know that there is a connection, but the probabilities are that there is some difficulty.

It may be the result of experiences with your own mother, or the result of early experiences with women, it may be that even your father enters into the picture in some way. Regardless of how this thing started, regardless of what anxieties, what fears, what distrust, what hostilities may exist in your relationships with women, they have absolutely nothing to do with present-day facts. They have absolutely nothing to do with your wife. Eventually you will deal with life less on the basis of early associations, early conditionings, early fears, no matter what they may have been, and more on the basis of present-day reality. It's not really necessary to unearth or to examine everything about your early life to produce results. It is not essential to our task right at this moment. We're going to work on the assumption that there is some sort of anxiety, some sort of fear in relationship to women, but that it is not important to bring it out at this time. No matter what your associations were before, no matter what difficulties you had with your mother, or other women, no matter what fantasies you may have had when you were little, or what fears there were, they did happen in the past. They are not a part of your present life. You must dissociate them from your present life.

Let us assume now that you do go to bed with your wife with the idea of getting whatever pleasure you can out of it. I'm going to suggest that you gradually throw away the other motivations, that is performing and pleasing her. Assume that it makes no difference how long it takes, really assume that, and go into sexual relations as a means of pleasing yourself, of seeing what pleasure you can get out of it. The suggestions that I'm giving you now about fitness, and your own ability to control stiffness and rigidity, will continue to operate in other areas. And I'm going to extend that suggestion so that it will lend strength and capacity for erectiveness in your sexual functions.

You can, if you wish, try to isolate yourself from the fears no matter what they may have been, no mattter what they are. At the same time let yourself assume that it makes no difference how long your penis remains erect. It may go down immediately, and if it does, you must get yourself to a state where you don't care. It may go down shortly after you insert it, and if it does, you must not care. It may continue in there for a minute, and then go down; it may continue for two minutes or three minutes or even more in a fully erect position. The important thing is you must insert it with the idea of seeing if there is any pleasure associated with intercourse. See if there is any pleasure associated with inserting it. Insert it with the idea that it makes no difference to your wife; it only makes a difference in how *you* feel. Finally, you must separate whatever anxieties or fears that exist in relationship to women, and in relationship to their sexual organs, from yourself. Just go ahead with the idea of getting as much fun out of sex as possible.

If you do all these things, you will notice that it will be possible to feel stiffness and rigidity in your penis that will enable you to function well. I'm going to give you another strong suggestion to that effect. You must now begin to dissociate, remove, whatever fears there may be. Don't concern yourself with them so much. It may not be necessary to look into them or to investigate them. If they're there, it will be increasingly possible to dissociate yourself from them, to remove them, to feel that they need not matter to you, that you can function and do well without them. I'm going to repeat the suggestion that the ability to conrol the stiffness in your penis will become more and more and more pronounced.

As you sit there, I'm going to ask you now to continue to sleep, continue to sleep, and again count slowly from one to five. At the count of five, you'll notice that your whole body will stiffen up and become rigid, firm, rigid, firm. As you sit there the rigidity will increase until I give you the command to loosen up. Count from one to five, and the whole body will stiffen up. It will be impossible for you to get out of the chair, and you continue to sleep until I give you the command to loosen up again.

Pt.   One, two, three, four, five.

Dr.   Even though you try to get up out of the chair, the harder you try, the stiffer you feel. In a moment, I'm going to talk to you again. In the meantime continue to sleep. (*Pause*) Now I'm going to count slowly from one to five, and at the count of five, the stiffness will be gone and you'll slowly awaken, slowly awaken. Then we'll talk some more. One, two, three, four, five. Open your eyes and wake up. How do you feel?

Pt. Drowsy.

Dr. I'm going to work with you in other areas besides the sexual one, because I think from your associations, that you have other problems like the ability to express aggressiveness and action. Do you have an opportunity in your work to express aggressiveness?

Pt. It doesn't call for a great deal of aggressiveness.

Dr. How about your relationships with your employees?

Pt. They're very good. They've always been good.

Dr. Good in a sense that they're congenial?

Pt. Yes.

Dr. It would be very, very helpful to you if you would be able to have an opportunity to express certain forceful feelings. It is important for you to practice being firm and holding your ground, being assertive and demonstrative. But this won't develop right away. It will take time. Do you have any athletic outlets?

Pt. Physical? No.

Dr. Physical exercises would be helpful, an outlet for forceful actions.

Pt. Yes.

Dr. Are you interested in any hobby? It would be good if you could get interested in something that would give you a chance at motor expression. Do you have any ideas you would like to talk about, any impressions or feelings?

Pt. No, but I have led a restrictive life.

Dr. The ability to express yourself forcefully in some sphere would be helpful to you.

Pt. Yes, I can see that.

Dr. Because you have led too restricted an existence.

Pt. That's right.

Dr. A passive kind of life.

Pt. True.

Dr. It's a little difficult to know exactly in what area your interests may lie. For instance, I knew a man who wasn't at all aware of the fact that he was inhibiting his aggression. He believed he was being civilized in hardly moving a muscle.

Pt. Yes?

Dr. And so I asked him why he didn't take up a hobby. He replied, "Well, what hobby?" We worked and we worked on this,

and finally he took up fencing. He was terrified the first few
times that he might hurt somebody. Well, it took effort and
courage to go ahead. He began seeing that he didn't kill anybody in fencing, and he got rid of a lot of pent-up aggression
within him. I don't know what hobby you might find interesting,
but something like that would be extremely helpful.

Pt.   I was thinking about golf.

Dr.   Even golf, you could just take a good lusty swing at the
ball, even get mad at it.

Pt.   (*Laughs*) Well, that's true, I don't get mad often enough.

Dr.   Try it, even if it's only a ball you get mad at. Wallop it as
hard as you can.

Pt.   I will.

Dr.   Get the aggression out of your system. Do you play golf now?

Pt.   No, but I will. I can see what you mean.

FIFTH SESSION (APRIL 10)

*The patient has been able to recognize his lack of aggression as
a problem. He has made an important gain, feeling for the first
time sensations in his penis during intercourse. He apparently
has accepted the suggestion given him to regard sex relations as a
source of pleasure rather than as an arena in which he proves
himself. We discuss the flowing rather than the spurting character of his ejaculations and connect it to the use of the penis as
a urinary rather than sexual organ. In hypnosis strong persuasive
arguments are given him, and an attempt is made to remove
misconceptions about masturbation.*

Pt.   I couldn't help but feel last time I left the office riding on
the subway that we're on the right track. I mean what you had
said seemed just right home.

Dr.   Particularly in what respect?

Pt.   About the aggressiveness in me not being there.

Dr.   Do you have any ideas about that?

Pt.   No, I haven't.

Dr.   Have you been aware of this lack all along?

Pt.   Yes, I have been aware of that.

Dr.   How far back does it go?

Pt. Well, about ten years is all I can remember. I've reproached myself more or less for it during that time.

Dr. How?

Pt. To me it was symbolic of a certain weakness.

Dr. All right, we can work on that along with the other if you wish. Has anything else happened since I saw you last?

Pt. Yes, but there wasn't much difference in my sex relations.

Dr. There was no difference at all?

Pt. I think, though, I detected a difference in feeling there. In other words I wasn't as anxious to perform and do good. The tension was less.

Dr. Good.

Pt. Yes, the desire to succeed wasn't as strong as it generally is. Another interesting thing is that for the first time when I inserted my penis, I think I really detected a difference.

Dr. Are you sure of that?

Pt. Yes.

Dr. You didn't concentrate your attention on the performance.

Pt. Yes. Somehow the ultimate outcome wasn't as important as it generally is.

Dr. Did you have an ejaculation last night?

Pt. Yes.

Dr. Were you able to observe if the ejaculation was a spurting ejaculation or a flowing one?

Pt. Well, I don't recall.

Dr. Did you note any muscular spasms as you ejaculated?

Pt. No, no.

Dr. It was just sort of like urinating?

Pt. That's right.

Dr. Well, it will be interesting to follow this along. When you masturbate is it a flowing or spurting ejaculation?

Pt. No, that's a spurt.

Dr. There's a difference, then. Now, do you recall any urinary fantasies or urinary activities as a child?

Pt. No, none of that kind, none at all.

Dr. There was never any such thing as bed wetting?

Pt. No, no.

Dr. Any such thing as noticing a little girl urinate?

Pt. No, no, nothing like that.

Dr. There is a difference in the two types of ejaculation.

Pt. I noticed that.

Dr. The flowing off may remind you of the urinary function.

Pt. It does.

Dr. And the absence of sensation in inserting the penis may be referable to the fact that the penis is not used as a sexual organ, but rather as a urinary organ.

Pt. I see.

Dr. I want you to concentrate on your feelings in your penis, on the ideas that came to you in intercourse. I want you to get as much pleasure out of the feeling of intercourse as possible.

Pt. That's right.

Dr. It is necessary to retrain your entire attitude toward sex and the sex act.

Pt. Yes.

Dr. This can be done. You must recast your attitudes so sex comes to have pleasure values for you. Now I want you to go to sleep. I'd like to have you lean back now and watch your hands. Just keep gazing at your hand, breathe deeply and then slowly begin to feel yourself getting drowsy, and then your hand will begin to get light. It must begin to move a little bit, the space between the fingers will widen and you'll begin to notice that the hand will start lifting up slowly, rising, and lifting, right up towards your face. As it rises and lifts up towards your face, you get sleepier and sleepier until finally you go to sleep. Your hand will continue to rise and lift. You get sleepier and sleepier and sleepier, and the hand will rise towards your face, until it touches your face. When it touches your face, you will be asleep, deeply asleep. You will get drowsy, you'll breathe deeply, you'll go to sleep. Your hand touches your face now. Breathe in deeply. Sleep; lean back and go to sleep. In a moment I'll talk to you, and you will be still more deeply asleep. (*Pause*)

I'm going to suggest to you that as you sit there, you, yourself, count from one to five, and at the count of five, you'll be cognizant of a stiffness and rigidity in your fingers, in your hand, in your arm, that makes the hand stretch itself out, and the arm will stretch itself out, this way. Go ahead, start counting now. Count from one to five.

(An attempt is made here to get the patient to participate as much as possible in the therapeutic process in order that he begin to express more aggressiveness.)

Pt. One, two, three, four, five.

Dr. So that the arm becomes stiff, and even though you try to relax it, even though you try with all your might to move it, the harder you try the stiffer and heavier it becomes. Do you notice that?

Pt. Yes.

Dr. Do you notice that even when you try to make it relax and become soft, it's stiff and outstretched, hard and rigid?

Pt. Yes.

Dr. Now as you sit there, I'm going to stroke this arm again and only as I count from one to five will it become soft and come down. One, two, three, four, five. Now it comes down. Good. Sleep deeply. *(Pause)*

As you sit there, I'm going to ask you to visualize that scene in the theater where you noticed action. The last time you saw that scene the movement on the stage was extremely passive, people were sitting or standing. There was very little movement. All that is indicative of the lack of aggressiveness, the lack of assertiveness, the lack of movement in your life, the lack of push, the lack of masculine forcefulness. I would like to have you look upon the stage in your imagination now, and notice before you a picture of real forcefulness, of activity, of movement. I want you to notice that and as soon as you see that tell me about it. See if you can visualize and feel a scene of movement and forcefulness.

Pt. Someone dancing, a man and woman.

Dr. Now as you sit there, I want to see if you can visualize yourself in an aggressive role. Visualize yourself in the most aggressive role that you can possibly bring to your mind. As soon as you get a fantasy of that kind, tell me about it without waking up.

Pt. Swimming in a championship contest.

Dr. Did you visualize yourself swimming in a championship contest?

Pt. Yes.

Dr. Good. Now a problem that we have to tackle that's bound up with and associated with premature ejaculation is the idea of masculine forcefulness. It's necessary for you to bring out this material and see the significance of how far back it goes, and then take certain active steps with my help toward an entirely new orientation in regard to people, life, yourself and your own impulses, aggressive and sexual. As a child were you an aggressive child?

Pt. No.

Dr. Did you get into fights with the older boys?

Pt. Rarely.

Dr. How did you make out in those fights you got in?

Pt. Same as average, winning, sometimes losing. I tried to avoid any kind of trouble. I was afraid.

Dr. What happened to you that made you become so passive? Something occurred that put the floodgates on your aggressiveness, forcefulness and strength. What did happen to you is possibly not known to you now. But perhaps you may be able to recapture it through the medium of dreams, either now or later in the future. Of course, it is not absolutely essential to get the cause, but it's very essential to correct the effect. But getting the origin may make it possible to correct the effect more rapidly. Even though you may not possibly have the desire to get to the origin of your problem, because of time or any other reason, you still will be able to correct the effect of lack of aggression and lack of forcefulness that has permeated your whole life. Now, as you sit there, do you know of any incident or any series of incidents that frightened you?

Pt. No.

Dr. Did anything happen to you that made you feel that being hostile, being assertive, being forceful, having push, was not the proper or desirable way to be?

Pt. No.

Dr. Nothing like that. You will become increasingly aware of how important this problem is to you. You will become more and more aware of the fact that there is something lacking in your life, which will make you want to cooperate with me in a plan I shall outline for you. The first part of the plan involves your relationships with your wife. There is nothing more disastrous to effective sexual functioning than to look upon it as an arena in which you must demonstrate your virility and masculinity. Sex is no place of display. It has a different purpose. It is a procreative function that has pleasure values. You must regard sex in terms of pleasure, not performance. For that reason again I'm going to give you a forceful suggestion that when you go to bed with your wife and want to have sex with her, that you do it on a basis of your wanting to see how much fun you can get out of it. There may, perhaps, be the feeling that you don't know whether you can have fun, but in spite of that a part of you will desire to have pleasure out of sexuality. And that part of you will grow and will undermine the other part.

If you have any anxiety at all about this, if you have any tension, if you have any fear, or if you have any reluctance about coming here, I will expect you to tell me about it because it's very important. Also I want you to tell me about all the sensations you feel when you insert your penis in the vagina, no matter what those sensations may be—constriction, tingling, feeling of oppression, pain, pleasure or whatever sensations you may have. Observe them and see what feelings come to you, pleasure feelings or other feelings. Again I'm going to suggest that less and less you will look upon sex as an arena of performance, and more and more you must regard it as a means of finding important values and pleasures for yourself. You must begin to regard sexuality as a source of pleasure and not as a means of displaying or proving yourself.

Let us now discuss the matter of your self-confidence. As a result of the work that you do with me here, you are going to find that you can become more assertive, more self-confident, and more active than you've ever been.

Before we go on further I should like to explore an area with you that may be important. I'm going to give you a suggestion that you begin to feel yourself getting small as you sit here, that you feel yourself going back in time, getting little, very little. Your head is getting little, your arms are getting little, your legs are getting tiny. Feel yourself getting tinier and tinier, and going back, back, back in time to a point, let us say, when you were six years of age. Let us say that you visualize yourself as a little boy of six. Listen to the clock ticking, so that as the clock ticks back, ticks the time far back, you get little, very little. And when you talk to me next, you will be a little boy, you will be six years of age. As soon as you feel yourself six, as soon as you feel yourself small, you will indicate it by your hand, your left hand, rising up about two inches. Feel yourself getting small, little, six years of age. As soon as you do, your hand will rise up and indicate that you feel like six. Everything will be as it was when you were six years of age. Your hand rises now. How old are you?

Pt.   Six.

Dr.   What grade are you in?

Pt.   Two-B.

Dr.   You must have skipped, how old were you when you started school?

Pt.   Five.

Dr.   Now as you sit there, do you know your teacher's name?

Pt.   No.

Dr.   How do you get along with the other kids?

Pt.   All right.

Dr.   Do they fight with you?

Pt.   No.

Dr.   Do you get mad at them?

Pt.   No.

Dr.   Do they ever get on your nerves?

Pt.   No.

Dr.   How do you get along with your mother?

Pt.   Well.

Dr.   And your father?

Pt.   Well.

Dr.   And with the other people in the family?

Pt.   Well.

Dr.   Has anybody ever picked on you or wanted to hit you?

Pt.   No.

Dr.   They didn't? You're not afraid to fight, are you?

Pt. No.

Dr. Good. Now you begin to get a little bit older, older. You're thirteen years of age. You're exactly thirteen years of age. You're thirteen. The next time I talk to you you'll be thirteen years of age. How old are you now?

Pt. Thirteen.

Dr. What grade are you in?

Pt. Junior High.

Dr. Do you like school?

Pt. Yes.

Dr. How do you get along with the kids?

Pt. Well.

Dr. Do you get into fights with them?

Pt. Occasionally.

Dr. Does anybody in particular pick on you?

Pt. No.

Dr. Whom do you fight with?

Pt. Boys.

Dr. Why?

Pt. Get in little arguments.

Dr. How do you get along with your mother?

Pt. Fine.

Dr. And father?

Pt. Fine.

Dr. Do they ever pick on you?

Pt. No.

Dr. How about masturbation? When did you start masturbating?

Pt. About ten.

Dr. Did anybody teach you masturbation?

Pt. No.

Dr. How did you learn it?

Pt. I don't know.

Dr. Can you see yourself masturbating now?

Pt. Yes.

Dr. Do you feel that any harm can come to you if you masturbate? What do you think about it?

Pt. I do.

Dr. Do you think it's wrong?

Pt.   Yes.

Dr.   What may happen to you?

Pt.   I don't know, it's just that it's wrong.

Dr.   Did anybody ever tell you it's bad?

Pt.   No.

Dr.   Well, how do you know it's wrong?

Pt.   It just doesn't seem right.

Dr.   As you sit there, I'm going to tell you that all youngsters masturbate. No physical harm will come to you. But if your own feeling about masturbation is that it can do you harm, your own fear of masturbation can create guilt feelings which may cause anxiety. As you sit there I'm going to tell you that whatever fears, whatever destructive feelings you have had about masturbation, you will eventually get over them. Nothing will happen to you.

Now I want you to go back, or forward, whichever it may be, to the first time you put your penis in a woman. And I want you to describe to me in great detail how it happened, all your feelings, all your fears, if there were any, all your ideas, everything, just as if you were living through it again. As soon as you feel yourself there, tell me all about it as if you were living through that experience again.

Pt.   I remember going into the room with a girl undressed.

Dr.   Who was the girl?

Pt.   I don't know, she was a prostitute the first time.

Dr.   Did you go with the other fellows?

Pt.   Just one other fellow.

Dr.   What sort of a girl is she?

Pt.   She was an attractive girl.

Dr.   Younger, older than you?

Pt.   Older.

Dr.   What happens now?

Pt.   Well, we got into bed. Of course I was very nervous.

Dr.   Did you have all your clothes off?

Pt.   Ah, yes.

Dr.   Did she?

Pt.   Yes.

Dr.   And then what did she do, what did you do?

Pt.   Well, then we had intercourse.

Dr. What happened?

Pt. Well, I don't remember exactly the length of time before I ejaculated. I can't remember that. But I think it was very shortly.

Dr. Were you excited?

Pt. Yes.

Dr. And what happened directly afterwards? I'm interested in your thoughts, your ideas about that.

Pt. Well, I got dressed and left. I repeated it several times after.

Dr. That first time, how did you feel about it? Did you feel that it was or wasn't all right?

Pt. No, I felt it was all right. Being there I just felt that the act itself wasn't right. That is, I wasn't successful with it. Because I remember that I was with a friend of mine, and we occupied two separate rooms. I had gotten out so much sooner than he, and I was sitting and waiting for him in the ante room, and I felt that it was wrong to be through so much faster than he.

Dr. Were you ashamed of yourself?

Pt. Well, yes.

Dr. Did you feel that you weren't as good as he was?

Pt. That's right.

Dr. Do you feel that ejaculating prematurely makes you less of a man than other men?

Pt. Yes.

Dr. What happened after that? Did you go back to the same girl?

Pt. Once or twice after that.

Dr. And what happened?

Pt. The same thing.

Dr. Was there any fear of this girl at all? Or disgust with her?

Pt. No, no.

Dr. I see. As you sit there return to your present age. (*Pause*) It seems to me that we have a clue to what may be the basic problem here. There are doubts about your masculinity, some doubts about your aggressiveness, some doubts about yourself in comparison to other men. You have, for some reason, unfavorably compared yourself to other men, and that unfortunate comparison has influenced you and caused you to use a symbol wrongly. That is, you believe that you are less of a man than other men because you ejaculate prematurely. That is a wrong concept because basically you are a masculine person. It's only a misinterpretation of facts that has caused you to perform in this way. You are not impotent, and you are not unmasculine. You are a masculine person, and you must begin to exercise aggressiveness and build up a concept of your own aggressive activity. Your own feeling of masculinity in your relationship to others will finally spread to the sexual sphere also. I'm going to give you a strong suggestion to that effect. From the moment you leave here, you must begin to plan little actions that are aggressive in nature, no matter what they may be. It may be certain things that you do in your work. It may be certain things that you do in relationship to other people. It may be in the field of hobbies or activities. Whatever they are, before you come back next time, I want you to have done something that demonstrates a display of aggressiveness. Not destructive, but active and assertive aggressiveness. You understand me?

Pt.   Yes.

Dr.   It's extremely necessary that we build this thing up to a point where you can exercise your aggressiveness, because that's completely bound up with your whole concept of yourself and also your sexual functioning. Do you see that?

Pt.   Yes.

Dr.   Good. Continue to sleep now. In a moment I will wake you up and talk to you again. (*Pause*) And now slowly your eyes will open as I count to five. It makes no difference whether you remember or do not remember what is said here, you still will feel a compulsion to abide by the suggestions that I've given you. One, two, three, four, five. Wake up. . . . How do you feel?

Pt.   All right.

Dr.   Feel relaxed? How have you been sleeping?

Pt.   Well, I was always a good sleeper, but I think I have been sleeping better in the past week.

Dr.   You have relaxed better?

Pt.   Yes.

Dr.   Good. The things I have suggested to you are apt to create some tension and anxiety. There are reasons why you have inhibited yourself. The reason our efforts should be successful is that as a kid you were aggressive. You were forceful and expressive and then something happened to you that blocked you. I have an idea that it is bound up with masturbation and with fears that through masturbatory activities you had done yourself some irreparable harm.

Pt. Yes.

Dr. And there may have been an idea about masturbation that you should be more retiring than others because you might not be able to hold your own.

Pt. That's right. There was something very secretive about it to begin with. As a result of that I was perhaps a little more retiring.

Dr. Yes, and it is important to exercise aggressiveness. Whatever you do to express your own aggressiveness isn't so important as long as you do it. If you experience a little tension or anxiety about it, we'll discuss it. We'll try to overcome it so that eventually you'll be able to feel more and more expressive, aggressive, assertive, and more self-confident. You will be able to express yourself in all fields of action better, including your sexual activity. But there again the urgency of performing must be put down. The pleasure values are the important things here.

SIXTH SESSION (APRIL 17)

The patient has noticed that even though he ejaculated prematurely, pleasure sensations continue to be present in his penis, and the character of the ejaculation has become spasmodic instead of flowing. Further persuasive and reeducational suggestions are given him under hypnosis in the attempt to restore his sexual functioning. He evidences no desire to probe more deeply into his lack of aggressiveness and other character defects.

Pt. I'm sorry I had to miss the last session, but something bad has been happening to the entire business world. Our firm is feeling the slump and I had to stay in the office. The bottom has fallen out of the market.

Dr. How about your personal problems?

Pt. In spite of myself, I feel I'm just racing against time. I mean this is something I should have undertaken a long time ago.

Dr. Well, but now look, the urgency is part of your problem.

Pt. I see.

Dr. And what have you done about it? What has occurred?

Pt. Not much of a change other than I don't feel as keenly about it as I did another time. In other words, the idea of performance and disappointment of failure, I mean, it doesn't play as big a part.

Dr. It's important not to let the challenge element of it get you.

Pt. I see.

Dr. Now, in your own observance of your sexual feelings, what has happened there?

Pt. Well, there too, I found a slight change insofar as the sex act itself is concerned. Several weeks back my primary interest was being successful in the act. Now I seem to be getting more pleasure out of it.

Dr. But still the thing that disturbs you is a sense of frustration.

Pt. Exactly.

Dr. And perhaps a hectic anxiety that this next time it's going to be successful.

Pt. I can't seem to overcome that. I try to fight it but I can't.

Dr. I will just keep bringing it to your attention over and over again, because understanding is the thing that will help you. You just can't look upon it as a challenge. Sex is not meant as a challenge.

Pt. Yes, I understand.

Dr. All right, so that you begin to notice that you could get certain more pleasure out of sex?

Pt. That's right.

Dr. What precisely happens as you begin sex play now? How long after you start sex play do you insert?

Pt. I should say about ten to fifteen minutes.

Dr. Now does your wife have an orgasm?

Pt. No, but if I continue playing with her she does, as I did on one or two occasions.

Dr. Does that make you feel better?

Pt. Somewhat.

Dr. When you insert, what sensations have you noticed?

Pt. Well, the sensation is the feeling of having inserted. Prior to coming here I mean, my mind wasn't . . . I mean it was just that one thing, and I actually didn't feel anything, but now I get more feeling.

Dr. You get more feelings in your penis?

Pt. That's right.

Dr. Good, that's what I've been wanting you to see. That you can concentrate your attention on sensations and feel it's a pleasurable experience.

Pt. That's right.

Dr. Do you feel the orgasm when it comes?

Pt. That's right and last time for the first time it was spasmodic.

Dr. Spasmodic?

Pt. Yes, yes.

Dr. I see, it isn't a flowing?

Pt. No, no.

Dr. That's a great deal of progress.

Pt. Yes.

Dr. Now again we're going to work on the element of considering sex a source of pleasure and less a challenge. In addition we must work on the business of expressing your assertiveness, your aggressiveness, your forcefulness in other areas. Have you had a chance, the opportunity, to work at this forcefulness of expression?

Pt. Yes, in one or two instances I found that I had been more forceful. In business I found that I'm a little more assertive, a little more forceful in some of the enterprises and dealings with problems that come up. But I don't know, it may be due to the conditions of business today. I mean this rapid change. But in general I think, due to our meetings, there is appearing a little more forcefulness. I do feel a little more that way.

Dr. Very good, and you've got to continue that because that's terribly essential, very vital. Supposing you lean back in your chair now. Would you be more comfortable if you'd lie down?

Pt. No.

Dr. Just lean back in your chair, put your hands down and this time I want to have you very rapidly begin to feel yourself sinking into a deep, restful, relaxed, comfortable sleep. And as you do your hand, your right hand, will rise and lift, lift, slowly rise, just like that, right up to your face. And when it touches your face, you'll feel drowsy and tired, and sleepy, very sleepy, and drowsy and tired. The hand keeps rising and lifting, and you get sleepier and sleepier, from your head right down to your feet. Tired and drowsy and sleepy; you go into a deep sleep. Begin to sleep now, go into a sleep.

Now, as you sit there, I'm going to stroke your arm and the arm is going to start feeling heavy, heavy just like lead. Good . . . now go to sleep deeper and I'll soon talk to you. (*Pause*)

You have developed certain habit patterns and fears that are affecting your functioning. Your functioning has been impaired in several areas, mostly in the area of aggressive action and forcefulness, and in the area of your feelings of masculinity. Very fortunately you happen to be a masculine person and your aggressiveness has not been squashed. It has merely been snowed under. It's a matter of removing the restraints and the inhibitions. Then you will go forward. If it were true that your masculinity was crushed completely, you would not be able to have an erection as frequently as you do. Therefore your problem is not like the problem of a person with impotency, because you do have erections when you make love to your wife. Something happens to you as you insert that makes you feel as if you are not masculine.

We are going to work on the two areas. We're going to work on the area of your assertiveness, your forcefulness, your ability to express activity in your relationships with people and in your attitudes toward life. And then we're going to work more specifically on your sexual impulse. We're going to work at it until you overcome it.

I am going to suggest to you that you will overcome it in spite of any doubts, in spite of any fears that may come up. You are going to overcome this problem of premature ejaculation, and you're going to be able to function in a perfectly normal manner. You may doubt it, you may have fears about it; but the doubt and fears are merely products of your own emotional chaos. They will not deter you; you will, you must overcome the problem. You can, and you will.

I'm going to ask you to visualize certain things for me, and to tell them to me as you sit there with your eyes closed and in a drowsy state. I'm going to give you certain suggestions. I want you to start dreaming. The immediate feeling may be that you can't dream. That again is merely a block, an inhibition. You can dream, and if there is nothing more than just visualizing something, visualize it and tell it to me. As a last resort you may actually picture yourself in a theater looking up at a stage noticing actions in front of you just as if you were looking at a play. But whatever method you utilize, it's necessary for you to dream or fantasy things so we can make progress faster.

I am going to ask you now to dream about or to visualize something that arouses you sexually, something that is intensely stimulating to you sexually. No matter what it may be, I want you to have a sexual fantasy or a dream about something that is intensely exciting sexually for you. No matter what it may be, have that dream or fantasy and then tell me about it without waking up. (*Pause*)

Pt. A man and a woman walking into a hotel room, both undressing and lying on the bed. The man starts making love to the woman. They are both nude. He starts with kissing her, fondling her, holding her breasts. That excites him when he holds her breasts.

Dr. All right, now I'm going to ask you to have another dream or fantasy, and this time it has to do with something very fearful, something frightening. No matter whatever connection there may be, even though it's a remote one, tell me about it without waking up.

Pt. I had a dream of walking into a room, noticing a man or woman about to leap from a window.

Dr. Now I'm going to give you another suggestion and that has something to do with the thing that you had previously been dreaming about. I'm going to give you the suggestion to repeat that fantasy, to visualize a man making love to a woman, fondling her breasts, becoming intensely stimulated. Visualize the man having an erection and then going through the process of having intercourse. Now I want you to imagine that it takes place and as you visualize or fantasy or dream it, this arm over here will slowly lift up and become stiff and rigid; and it will remain that way so long as the man in the dream has an erection. The moment you see him losing his erection this arm will begin to loosen up, lose its rigidity and come down. I want you to fantasy that scene and be stimulated sexually. As you do notice his penis

become erect, automatically and without any effort your arm
will stiffen up, straight out in front of you, and will remain that
way so long as the man has an erect penis. Go ahead. As soon as
the penis no longer is erect the arm will drop down. (*Patient's arm
stiffens and then relaxes.*) Now I notice by actual time that this
took a minute and five seconds. Can you describe what happened
in your fantasy?

Pt. Well, there was an erection, the man inserted and remained
that way for that length of time.

Dr. Yes, a minute and five seconds. Now have you ever timed
how long your penis remains erect in the vagina?

Pt. No, maybe a few seconds.

Dr. Gradually that period will increase, gradually it will increase and the time that you have a full erection will become
longer and longer and longer. It will increase to a point where
it eventually will become normal. Now the normal period is as
you know between three minutes and ten minutes. I'm going to
give you a suggestion that gradually you are going to feel in
control because you will be able to control the erectivity of your
penis. Whatever sensitivity exists will not force you to have
a premature ejaculation. You will be more concerned with the
pleasure you get out of sex than with the performance.

As you have sexual relations, I want you to keep in mind a
picture of yourself as a forceful person engaged in some forceful
act. I'm going to give you a suggestion now in which you visualize
yourself as a forceful person doing something forceful no matter
what that may be. I want you to visualize yourself doing something
forceful no matter what that may be. I want you to visualize
yourself as a forceful person doing something forceful. As soon
as you do that or dream it, tell me about it without waking up.
(*Pause*)

Pt. I had a dream about addressing a jury on the behalf of the
defendant.

Dr. And doing a good job?

Pt. Yes.

Dr. Good. I'm going to give you two suggestions. First, I want
you to practice being forceful and assertive in your business, in
your relations with people, because you realize this is important

for you. And, second, exercise force and assertiveness in your relationships with your wife. When you have sex next, I should like to have you observe the length of time that elapses from the time of insertion of the penis to the time that you withdraw. This may be a little difficult at first because you will feel challenged. The very time element is the thing that concerns you so much. So that looking at a clock may have certain panicky connotations for you. But you will overcome those panicky feelings; perhaps you may not even think of them. Observe the time from when you insert the penis to when you remove it.

Again I want you to feel that the pleasure function in sex is the primary concern. As you insert your penis, observe your feelings and sensations and do not be concerned with how long it lasts. Enjoy the act and orgasm. As you have sex, you can then visualize yourself as a forceful person; visualize yourself in a capacity of doing something forceful even though you may have to utilize a fantasy of being a forceful person. I want you to tell me what that fantasy is. Do not be concerned with the time even though you do want to know how long it lasts. Again I repeat, even though you feel obligated to regard sex as a challenge, you will be less and less concerned with it as a challenge and more as a pleasure function. Have you told your wife that you're coming to see me?

Pt. No.

Dr. How do you feel about telling her that you're doing something about yourself?

Pt. I'd rather not.

Dr. If you would rather not, it isn't necessary to tell her unless you, yourself, decide to do so. I'm going to ask you now slowly to start waking up as I count. At the count of five begin waking up slowly, open your eyes and wake up. When you wake up, you'll have a sense of relaxation. You must follow the suggestions that I've given you. You will even though you do not think about them or force yourself to do them. They will come about more and more automatically. I'm going to count from one to five, and at the count of five open your eyes and wake up. One, two, three, four, five. (*Patient opens his eyes.*) How do you feel?

Pt. All right.

Dr. Good. Let us discuss the business of telling your wife about your treatments. Do you feel that if you told her, she might not respect you?

Pt. Well, I guess that's it. Yes, I feel that if I did, I would have to more or less elaborate on the entire thing and my background and all. I don't care to do that.

Dr. You feel perhaps ashamed of it?

Pt. Somewhat, yes.

Dr. What parts of it?

Pt. Well, if I had to go into detail about the masturbatory period and the whole thing it might not look right. I mean in that case the question might arise why hadn't I told her about this sooner?

Dr. Actually it's your worry and guilt that makes it seem so terrible a situation. Because there's nothing that you've gone through that is so unusual. All people go through early experiences of which they are fearful or ashamed. Our culture makes people feel guilty about sex. If you talk to your wife, you probably would find that she also felt guilt feelings about sex when she was little. It is not necessary to tell your wife unless you feel you want to. Now how has she reacted to you in the past few times you had sex?

Pt. Same way, very lovely, very understanding.

Dr. Yes?

Pt. Optimistic and all.

Dr. Well, you must not regard her optimism as tolerance, as if she's standing by and waiting for great things to happen.

Pt. That's right.

SEVENTH SESSION (APRIL 23)

The symptom of premature ejaculation is beginning to clear up. In addition the patient finds that he is more active and assertive in his interpersonal relationships. Another attempt is made to motivate him toward going more deeply into his personality difficulties and to swing him into a nondirective or analytic type of therapy. He continues to show resistance to this effort.

Dr. Well, how have things been with you?

Pt. Well, I noticed a slight improvement, a real improvement.

One thing I saw was I was a little, I'm not as tense and excitable as I was, and I also found a little improvement in the time element. I think it's increased somewhat.

Dr.   Have you actually timed it?

Pt.   Well, not that far, but mentally I've tried to recall the time, and I find there's an increase of almost half a minute to a minute.

Dr.   Well, that's fine.

Pt.   Yes, I thought so.

Dr.   That's very, very fine, but we're not satisfied with that only. It has to continue. Now altogether how much time would you say elapses in intercourse?

Pt.   Well, now it's close on, I should say, it's close on to a minute and a half.

Dr.   Well, that's more like it now. Now have you noticed anything about your ideas or thoughts during the process of intercourse?

Pt.   No, my thoughts are pretty much alike, the original form, that is the anxiety to be successful, but with less degree of tenseness.

Dr.   Without any great degree of urgency?

Pt.   Yes.

Dr.   Has your wife noticed any change?

Pt.   Yes she has, yes.

Dr.   What is the relationship between the two of you now? Does she know about your coming here?

Pt.   No, she doesn't, no.

Dr.   And you're not anxious to let her know?

Pt.   No, I'd rather not unless it was absolutely urgent.

Dr.   It is not urgent. If it is part of a problem that has to do with deep feelings toward her, we should understand it. For instance, I treated a man who had a problem of this sort and who was afraid to let his wife know that he came here for definite psychological reasons that were more important than the premature ejaculations. Until we clarified these reasons, his symptoms persisted.

Pt.   I see. Well, the actual reason, I suppose, is that it would presuppose that I was aware of this thing long, long before. Perhaps I should have consulted her about it prior to asking her to marry me. And, insofar as I did not, an impression of my neglect might arise, and I would feel at a loss for an answer. Other than to say that I did consult a physician who said it was perfectly all right to marry, other than that, I mean, I couldn't very well explain it.

Dr. How much does she know about how long this thing has been going on?

Pt. Only from the day of our marriage.

Dr. Well, it's all right for her not to know anything more about it if you do not want to tell her. It isn't a really spectacular or permanent problem; believe me when I tell you that. The sexual difficulty is not the most significant thing compared to the overall picture. As a matter of fact you will notice that your sexual life will improve as you get confidence in your ability to go ahead and not look upon sex as a performance, but as a source of enjoyment. If you are not too urgent about it, you'll find this thing will straighten out. Perhaps then you will want to work more on your deeper personality problems.

Pt. Well, I see the change from day to day. Of course I'm still eager to have it one hundred percent normal, because almost normal is not enough, I mean.

Dr. That eagerness is understandable, but if you can just get yourself into a frame of mind where it's not too urgent or important, it will continue to improve. There is nothing more that blocks a person's effectiveness than to feel challenged and incapable of meeting the challenge. It's like a man I knew, who illustrates how feeling challenged and comparing himself unfavorably with others destroyed his sexual capacities. He was functioning well sexually until he met a woman he believed was his ideal. He married her and after that found himself to be a little frightened and couldn't have an erection. He got very panicky and the next time he tried it, success was so important to him that he couldn't have an erection. He was in a state of terror. It turned out that his wife's approach to him was one of making demands, and instead of reassuring him she began to compare him unfavorably with her previous husband. Thereafter he couldn't function, and the more upset he became, the less the possibilities of success. His sexual problem was, like others, the result of a difficulty in relationships and self-evaluation. I told him exactly the same thing that I told you: "Look, just don't get panicky, don't look upon sex as a challenge. If you can straighten out your relations with your wife, and realize that because you feel you are not as good as her first husband sexually, and if you can stop feeling challenged and have sex for pleasure, you will overcome your impotency." He, too, was able to correct his sex problem, but it was necessary later to work on why he permitted himself to be thrown by a statement of his wife. That took a longer time. The sexual function is one of the first affected by a relationship problem.

Pt. I see. A friend of mine told me recently that he knew of one fellow who had suffered from the same thing and took a series of injections and said it seemed to help him.

Dr. Some types of impotency are glandular and the treatment is injection with testosterone.

Pt. I see.

Dr. But your type of problem is psychological, not physical. Testosterone would contribute little. If I thought it would be helpful, you'd get it.

Pt. Yes.

Dr. What is necessary is building up your own confidence in yourself, of not being too much concerned with whether you succeed or fail. What about your activity in other areas—your aggressiveness, your outspokenness, your forcefulnss?

Pt. Well, too, I found that it improved since last week, since the several times we spoke about it. There, too, as I think I said before, I don't know whether it's the condition that brings it about, or because the business picture has changed so completely that out of necessity I may find that I'm a little more aggressive.

Dr. Whatever the cause, it doesn't matter so long as you go ahead.

Pt. Well, I do find I'm a little more assertive. There's no question about it.

Dr. Fine. Did you have any dreams since I saw you last?

Pt. Yes, I did some, but they've been so vague that the next day I tried to recall them and couldn't very well.

Dr. You can't remember any of them?

Pt.   No, but there have been some.

Dr.   The important thing now is to go along in the same direction of putting yourself in a position where you are outspoken and effective in what you do.

Pt.   Yes.

Dr.   If anything happens to your business in the impending recession, how do you believe you will react?

Pt.   Well, that's not affecting me as far as my condition is concerned. This is so much more important to me. I mean we've been through good times and bad times. It's a cycle and I'm accustomed to it. It's not having too great an effect on me. This thing is really paramount.

Dr.   It is paramount, but you're beginning to see your way clear. You're improving because you actually have gotten hold of some of the causes now. You can see that it's on the basis of your own underevaluation of yourself, the challenge to your masculinity. Once you overcome this, there isn't any real reason why you just can't barge ahead, go forward. We have spoken about the origins of this thing and how far back it goes. A person carries over with him in his present-day functioning, attitudes and feeling that started when he was very little. And unconsciously without even knowing it, these become a pattern that dominates the person's life. It's necessary to challenge that pattern. Ask yourself if you still are functioning like a little boy functioning under the aegis of a mother who is directing you, and a father who is supervising or condemning you. It's necessary to take stock of yourself.

Pt.   That's right.

Dr.   You're grown up now and life is an entirely different proposition than when you were little. It may be important to inquire psychologically into yourself, to see the disparity between what you were and what you are. You're not living in the past now. I think that if your relations with your wife become perfectly all right to you, you may be happier than you've ever been in all your life. But you'll continue to be happier if you get to the source of your trouble. That will require more treatment and a different approach, more or less analytic.

Pt.   Certainly I'm very much happier now than I was a month ago, not through any difference or attitude on my wife's part. It's just that I have more confidence now that this thing will work out, where a month ago I was very scared, very panicky. Today I am not. Of course a great deal of that is due to her very loving-ness and considerateness. I mean, she seems to make very light of it. She has all the patience in the world, and she is very confi-dent that in time this will wear off and everything will be fine. She's very happy under the conditions as they are today, so natu-rally if everything gets well, so much the better.

Dr. You feel she's happy with you now?

Pt. Well, that gets me to thinking sometimes. Is it so, or is she trying to ease my mind and just trying to be nice? Because after all a woman does have to be satisfied, she gets around from time to time, and that's all there is to it.

Dr. It is true that woman needs sexual gratification, but the very fact that you love her and she feels loved, and makes a physi-cal contact in being in your arms, can be gratifying, appeasing and satisfying.

Pt. That's what she says.

Dr. To repeat, the sexual act to you should not be associated with running a hundred-yard dash in nine seconds flat. It should rather be an experience that is an act of pleasure. And you find that you can do that right now?

Pt. Yes, I do.

Dr. You notice a change in your sexual responses?

Pt. That's right.

Dr. All right, supposing you lean back and go to sleep. Watch your hand, keep gazing at it; you'll notice that it will slowly get light, will rise and lift straight up in the air. As it approaches your face, you'll get drowsier and drowsier, and your eyes will get heavier and heavier until they go to sleep, until they shut. And as the hand rises, a sense of sleepiness will creep over you from your head down to your feet, and you will go into a deep, restful, relaxed, comfortable sleep. Your hand rises, goes up, up, straight up, up towards your face, and you get drowsier and drowsier. Now lean your head against your hand and rest and sleep for about a few minutes, and at the end of that time I'm going to talk to you again, and you'll be still more deeply asleep. (*Pause*)

Both in your work here with me while you are asleep, and in your actions outside, you will develop a certain sense of mastery, of confidence and assertiveness such as you probably have never known before. This will lead to an entirely different attitude towards yourself and towards your functions, including your sexual functions.

You have gone through experiences with me that have demonstrated to you the power of your own will and the effect that thinking and conceptualizing through suggestion has upon your physical functions. I'm going to ask you now to visualize that same scene where you feel sexually aroused, where you visualize something that stimulates you sexually. As you do, your left arm will gradually rise and become stiff, so stiff that it will be impossible for you to move it. It will become so stiff and rigid, it will be impossible for you to budge it. Now visualize a scene that is sexually arousing, stimulating, and as soon as you do, your arm will become so stiff and rigid that it will be impossible for you to budge it. Your arm is outstretched in front of you now; it's rigid and it's firm and stiff and it's going to remain that way until I give you the command to bring it down. . . .

Now slowly the arm comes down, right down to the thigh, and you're going to be able to feel in better control of your own functions including your sexual functions. You'll notice that your assertiveness will increase within yourself, but in addition you will have a desire to inquire more deeply into your problems, so that you can improve most successfully. You will find that the sexual act is not one in which you feel challenged, but one in which you can get pleasure. Your erection will get more vigorous and will remain with you, and the length of time it persists will continue to improve.

You will notice that the sex act will last longer and longer as you get confidence in yourself. This does not necessarily mean that you have to be consistent in the upswing. Perhaps you will be, but there may be times when, for certain emotional reasons, there may be a temporary slipback. That means nothing, and I want you to be in a position where you pay no attention to having an ejaculation prematurely. Do not get panicky about it because next time it will probably be better. Look upon sex less and less as a challenge, and more and more as a source of pleasure, and you will find that you do well, and will be able to have normal, good, sexual relations.

Even more important is that you reorient yourself in your attitudes towards people, towards yourself and towards life and that you feel that you can be capable of an aggressive, demonstrative stand in the world. The latter will probably require deeper therapy.

Now I'm going to ask you to repeat for me that scene in which you go into a theater, sit down, look up at the stage and notice that the curtain opens and you see action on the stage. You see something on the stage. Whatever it is, I want you to visualize it vividly, and as soon as you do, raise your left hand which will indicate to me that you've seen the scene on the stage. (*Patient raises his hand.*) Now bring your hand down and tell me what you saw on the stage.

Pt. There's a courtroom scene with a judge and an attorney addressing a jury.

Dr. On any particular issue? Or is he just addressing the jury?

Pt. Well, he's addressing the jury in defense of a murder defendant.

Dr. I see. Continue to sleep, continue to sleep, continue to sleep. Breathe in deeply now, very deeply. I'm going to ask you to visualize another thing with me. Visualize yourself walking along the street with me. We enter a churchyard and we notice, right in front of us, a tall church steeple. You look at the church steeple, and you notice that there is a bell, and you notice the bell moving. As soon as you get the impression of the bell moving, you hear the bell clanging or get an impression of it clanging. Indicate this by your hand rising up just about an inch. (*Patient's hand rises.*) Good, now bring your hand down.

As you sit there again, I'm going to reinforce the suggestion that I've given you. Basically you are a fairly well integrated person, you can function fairly effectively as you are, but you must not be satisfied with the way you're functioning because you have the potentiality and the capacity to do better, to do more for yourself. You are not taking advantage of your own abilities and capacities, you are not doing what you're capable of doing yet, but you're getting there. You're seeing more and more clearly that you've been stymied, that as a result of what has happened to you before, you have restricted yourself and your capacities. You are going to be able, as you sit there, to envisage a life for yourself of far greater possibilities.

One of the most important steps that you took was to get married. It showed that you were not satisfied to live a celibate life, a life in which you would operate as if you were damaged. I don't know how you got the misconception about masturbation, but it really did not injure you physically. You have done nothing, absolutely nothing, of which you need be ashamed. Some children get the idea that when they do something that's pleasurable, of which the parents perhaps do not approve, that it's tantamount to being a murderer. You are not an evil person and never were. But you yielded too much to the forces of conscience, you yielded too much to the demands you imagined society imposed on you. Those were misconceptions. Fortunately you were able to correct those misconceptions before you got too old, before you could not enjoy yourself. It's up to you now to go forward further, to live a much more happy and integrated life than you've ever lived before. You're making steps in that direction and you must continue to make steps. You're going to be happier and happier as days go by, and you will improve in every area including the sexual area.

I want you to sit there for a few minutes and then I'll wake you up. (*Pause*) Now as you sit there, I'm slowly going to ask you to begin awakening. First, I'm going to count from one to five, and at the count of five, you'll slowly open your eyes and then wake up. One, two, three, four, five. Slowly open your eyes. (*Patient opens his eyes.*) We've gone through what I think is the fundamental basis of this symptom of yours, what caused it and how it affects you now, don't you think so?

Pt. Yes, I do.

Dr. So that now it's a matter of going deeper to understand how your personality problems started and how they affect you now. You'll notice that there may be tendencies for you to feel discouraged, for you to feel that you are going backward. But this will be temporary and you'll be able to snap out of it.

Pt. I did feel hopeless about it, but I don't now.

Dr. Good.

EIGHTH SESSION (MAY 6)

The patient missed several sessions ostensibly because of business emergencies. Actually as he began to function well sexually, he saw no further reason for continuing, since his motivation for therapy was merely the desire to have successful sexual relations. Resistance apparently was created by suggestions to probe deeper into his problems, which probing he undoubtedly regarded as a threat to his character defenses. He reports a definite improvement in his sexual life, his premature ejaculations no longer interfering with successful intercourse.

Dr. It's been a long time since I saw you.

Pt. Yes.

Dr. How are things?

Pt. Very nice.

Dr. I see.

Pt. Progressing very nicely. It's just been about a week that improvement is really marked. There's been a complete change in the time element.

Dr. How long do you go in intercourse?

Pt. Well, last time I went very long. About a week ago, for the first time in intercourse, I found that the time element was extended to a considerable degree. By that I mean, it was at least three minutes. But as elated as I was over that experience, it turned out to be an unfortunate one in this respect. I imagine prior to that my wife probably wasn't sufficiently aroused to make any particular difference as to the length of time, but in this case, having lasted that length of time, she naturally was aroused to a pitch where she was almost ready for an orgasm, and I couldn't stay with her and she was quite upset about it. Of course the next day everything had been forgotten and it was all over. But it had somewhat of an effect on me. As I say, ordinarily I would have been very elated over the fact that the time was extended to what it was, but having let her down that way had an effect on me. So much so that the next night I just wasn't good for anything. I got an erection and I lost it, and I got it back again. It was a question of a minute and it was all gone. And then after that it came back again better than before, and has been going that way for over a week now. Say about five days I have had a normal erection and a normal insertion. I find that without any difficulty it will last a good number of minutes. And that idea is just naturally leaving me as I go along, the idea that it's just a performance. The confidence is instilled, I mean I feel in other words today that now there is no reason that I have to prove myself. I do not see how I can improve further.

Dr. It's just a matter of deciding how far you want to go. You have shown a symptomatic improvement.

Pt. Great thing, to me a tremendous thing.

Dr. You're not taking too seriously your wife's being disconcerted last week?

Pt. Fortunately I married the type of girl she is. She's very sweet, she's very lovely. As I say it was just momentary, not that she said anything, but that feeling naturally had to be there. Of course the next day it was as though nothing had happened, which in itself made it a little easier for me. Yes, she's had orgasms since then. Of course, she, too, feels the same way. I mean at that first experience, she probably didn't realize at the moment that the fact that I did improve to such an extent—all she could feel at that time was the feeling that . . . but I suppose today she realizes that step by step she's going to lead a normal life.

Dr. It's just a matter of time.

Pt. That's right.

Dr. You are functioning fairly well now?

Pt. That's right. Well, I feel today that if I can possibly extend that another minute or two at the most, it will be fine, nothing to worry about.

Dr. Well, there's no reason why you can't. But again you must be warned about the business that there may be setbacks. Have courage to go forward. It's discouraging to be set back for a little while, but it's nothing permanent.

Pt. Well, I'm very happy over the results I've enjoyed so far.

Dr. How about your own personal life?

Pt. Well, I don't know that it has been changing just as you stated. I mean I think I am a little more assertive, but I don't, ah, by that I mean, I really feel so good over this prospect, that I know at least that there's a chance that I will be all right. It's been proven that I have improved. I feel it. I know it's there. It's not my imagination, so naturally that in itself has given me a different feeling.

Dr. I see, how do you feel about coming back here? Do you feel that you have the understanding, and that you've got the drop on this thing so that you can proceed on your own? How do you feel?

Pt. I don't know.

Dr. Well, you can continue coming here and we can work more intensively at personality problems toward more assertiveness.

Pt. I suppose so.

Dr. But you have overcome one hurdle.

Pt. I see.

Dr. Just the feeling of self-confidence about this thing. . . .

Pt. That's sufficient.

Dr. That's sufficient?

Pt. In time you feel that it will improve as I go along?

Dr. It should.

Pt. Say, I think it's almost, I would say almost normal today. Now if I can only extend that a little then it would be normal.

Dr. We can continue until you feel that you've gone as far as you like in the sexual or any other area.

Pt. Yes.

Dr. And you seem to feel that you've gotten as much out of coming here as you can. Now in your contacts with people have you noticed any change?

Pt. Yes, I am a little more assertive, a little more forceful in small ways perhaps, but nevertheless it's sufficient so that I can detect a little change. With that, too, I am sure that it's due to the realization, I mean I think it is the, ah, due to our talks that I'm beginning to see that and act accordingly.

(At this point I decide to show the patient the Rorschach cards to see if any structural changes have occurred.)

Dr. I'm going to show you these cards again and I want you to tell me what you see again. This is the first card.

Pt. I see an eagle, the shape of an eagle.

Dr.   The whole thing?

Pt.   Yes.

Dr.   This is the second.

Pt.   I see a pair of little dogs. Their paws meeting. That's all.

Dr.   This is the third.

Pt.   Poodle dogs with their paws meeting. I can't seem to determine the position though.

Dr.   Turn it any way you wish.

Pt.   They seem to be standing on their hind legs.

Dr.   Who?

Pt.   These, the dogs. No more.

Dr.   Dogs standing on their hind legs. Where do you see the dogs? Oh, yes. This is the fourth.

Pt.   I can't determine it. The two animals running down the trunk of a tree? Maybe squirrels.

Dr.   Where do you see the two animals? Oh, inside.

Pt.   In there, yes, down the trunk of the tree.

Dr.   Down the trunk of the tree. Go ahead. This is the fifth one here.

Pt.   Looks like an animal. It seems to me like the shape of a sea gull or bat.

Dr.   This is the sixth.

Pt.   Fur pelt. A staff on top. That's all.

Dr.   This is the seventh.

Pt.   The top of this are some mythological figures of some kind on a wall.

Dr.   This is the eighth.

Pt.   Two animals perched on some mountain. A pair of lions. Don't seem to see more.

Dr.   All right, and that's the ninth one, there.

Pt.   This way there might be two buffaloes.

Dr.   Those green ones?

Pt.   Yes. I can't see anything else.

Dr.   That's the last one.

Pt.   It's a group of squirrels in trees, crabs, sea food.

   (*It will be seen that there is a slight, but no remarkable change in his responses.*)

Dr.   Fine. Now draw a picture of a man and a woman. (*There was practically no change in the crude drawings of the heads of a man and a woman as compared to the original drawings.*) As I explained to you once before, it is not merely the problem of your premature ejaculation, but rather that the premature ejaculation was the product of a lot of other things. Consequently you can benefit from treatments not only in terms of sexuality, but in the way you react towards other people and towards life in general. You have noticed a change in yourself other than sexual improvement.

Pt. Yes, definitely.

Dr. A stronger feeling about yourself.

Pt. That's right.

Dr. Good. How's the business?

Pt. Terrible.

Dr. So that is not the reason for your improvement.

Pt. No, no.

Dr. Fine. Now I'd like to have you sit back and go to sleep.

Pt. Yes, of course.

Dr. Put your hands down on your thighs, watch your fingers and begin to feel a sensation of lightness and drowsiness. (*Patient closes his eyes and sleeps.*) Now as you sit there I'm going to repeat to you what I've said before, and you will be able to integrate and absorb what I have to say to you and to utilize it in a constructive way for yourself.

The entire problem of your capacity to function in a sexual relationship, seems partially to have been produced by a misconception about the damage that you presumably did to yourself through masturbation. Actually no physical hurt was done; but much psychological damage. It's fear that is your enemy and nothing else. The fact that you continued to masturbate against your judgment made you feel like a hypocrite. This had a damaging effect upon your aggressiveness and activity.

Why you reacted the way you did depended on the kind of parents and upbringing you had. The fact that you had to be good in order to feel secure and loved to some extent hampered your activity, and froze your feelings in spite of yourself. You felt no right to be expressive or aggressive. But it hasn't really hurt you.

Fortunately your upbringing impaired but did not destroy you.

That's the important thing, it has not hurt you permanently. You have the seeds of everything it takes to function. You've been able to proceed to marriage; you are in love with your wife; you are able to derive pleasure out of sex. And your capacity to feel pleasure out of sex will increase. Again you must not look upon it as a marathon; you must regard it as a casual experience in which you can derive pleasure. Sex should not be used to prove that you're a man or that you're not a man. It must not be utilized for that purpose. Use sex as a source of pleasure for yourself. The urgency of performing perfectly will then vanish. You have noticed that as you've been less and less concerned with the urgency to have an erection for a long time, that you've succeeded better and better. You will continue to succeed better and better. Your sense of confidence will return and you will feel stronger and more capable, not only in terms of sexuality, but in terms of a capacity to take a stand in life, to engage in aggressive, productive activities.

As you sit here now, I am going to give you a strong suggestion that the gains you've shown up to this time will continue. Even if there are slip-backs, you must not be upset. The less concern you show, the better you will be able to function. Again I am going to repeat that when you engage in sexual relations, do it from the standpoint of pleasure and not from the standpoint of having to perform. A misconception may still be residual in you that there's something fundamentally wrong with your sexual organs. There is nothing fundamentally wrong with your sexual organs. It is your attitude that has been twisted by unfortunate early experiences. Your attitude will change, and you will get better and stronger. Perhaps you will decide to go deeper into your problems.

I am going to count now from one to five. At the count of five, open your eyes and wake up. One, two, three, four, five. (*Patient awakens.*) How do you feel?

Pt. Fine.

Dr. Now supposing we discuss your coming back for further treatments. How do you feel about this?

Pt. Maybe on the basis of once in two weeks we could accomplish something.

Dr. Would that be better for you?

Pt. Yes, it would be better because it's very difficult for me to get away.

Dr. At this particular period?

Pt. At this particular period, the business crisis and all.

Dr. All right, we can then continue on this basis. We could make it two weeks from today or sooner if you telephone.

Pt. Fine.

(This was the last session. Telephone messages from the patient indicated a consistent improvement. He was certain that he had conquered his sexual problem and that he was functioning in a normal manner. Because of this, and because he had no desire to probe deeper into his personality problem, he stopped treatments indicating that he might return at a later date.)

HYPNOSIS AND ALCOHOLISM

BY

DR. S. J. VAN PELT

By reason of its widespread social as well as individual consequences alcoholism has always presented a serious problem. The amiable drunkard so often portrayed in book, stage or screen stories is no object of amusement to his relatives in real life. Countless lives have been ruined, marriages broken up, careers spoilt and untold misery brought about by addiction to alcohol. The essential nature of the problem has remained obscure and alcoholism has been regarded variously as being simply a disease in itself, either bio-chemical or allergic in nature, or merely the symptom of an under-lying nervous disorder.

As may be expected when the exact nature of the condition is uncertain the treatments advocated have been both numerous and varied. These range from medical procedures, using drugs such as apomorphine, emetin and the recently discovered Antabuse, which make it impossible to take alcohol without unpleasant effects, to moral and religious influences exerted by the Church, Temperance Societies and groups such as "Alcoholics Anonymous."

Medical treatment usually means treatment in an institution in order to make sure that the patient carries out the treatment and has no access to alcohol. In addition some treatments are not with-out danger and cases of death have been reported during Antabuse therapy even in apparently healthy individuals.

Group therapy such as that employed by Alcoholics Anonymous means attendance at meetings of fellow sufferers where the alcoholic is urged and persuaded to refrain from drinking no matter how much he may desire to do so.

Institutional, and the latter treatment also to a lesser extent, carries a certain amount of stigma and the alcoholic is apt to regard himself as someone who is definitely outside the run of ordinary human beings. This suggestion, for reasons which we will see later, is not at all desirable.

All these treatments, mental, moral, religious or medical, have at least one thing in common, they can all claim a percentage of successes. It is by no means unknown for an alcoholic to "see the light" at a religious meeting and to give up drinking completely, while medical and psychotherapeutic measures have their quota of successes.

This fact, that all common methods of treating alcoholism have a percentage of successes, throws an interesting light on the possible nature of its cause. What relationship can there be between religious and medical methods of treatment? What becomes of the theory of biochemical and allergic origins of alcoholism when psychotherapeutic measures effect a cure? What in fact *does* happen to the confirmed drunkard who suddenly gives up alcohol for good? It is undeniable that cases of almost instantaneous cure do occur. In such cases the general conditions affecting the patient remain the same. His personal history, often of nervousness, anxiety and hardship, remains the same. Factors alleged to have influenced his downfall, social conditions, family troubles or financial worries, remain the same. Only one thing has changed—the patient's mind—and he thinks (and feels) "I have no desire for Alcohol," whereas before he thought, "I must have Alcohol." What can bring about such a radical change of mind often in the space of only a few minutes? Under what conditions do we find similar extraordinary changes?

Those familiar with hypnosis will be fully aware of the extraordinary mental changes which can be brought about in this condition. It is unfortunately a common experience to see completely sober people behaving like drunkards at the command of some stage hypnotist. Although such spectacles are completely unedifying and undesirable they serve to show the amazing changes which can be produced in a susceptible person. Stage hypnotists work only with highly susceptible subjects whom they deliberately select from volunteers by means of simple tests. Such people can be very deeply influenced and will often carry out the most complicated post-hypnotic suggestions.

Naturally, no responsible person would suggest such a thing, but it is highly likely that a deeply hypnotized person who could be persuaded to act like a drunkard would respond to a posthypnotic suggestion to the effect that he would desire alcohol. This would be all the more likely if he could be cleverly persuaded that "alcohol was good for him"—that he "needed alcohol to keep his strength up," etc.

We know that self-hypnosis is an established fact and that in people who can achieve this state the most remarkable effects such as anaesthesia can be obtained. Is it possible that alcoholism can be due to accidental self-hypnosis? How could this come about? When we examine the history of an alcoholic we can usually divide it into three stages.

First of all alcohol is taken for social reasons and the patient has the idea firmly fixed in his head that it is "the thing to do," that drinking makes him "one of the crowd," that drinking is "manly" or "sophisticated" and that people who do not drink are "queer" or "out of it."

Secondly there is nearly always a period of stress or strain when alcohol is taken in increasing amounts. During this period alcohol is regarded as a friend for it smooths over the difficulties and apparently makes life easier.

Finally in every alcoholic there comes a time when he suddenly realizes that he cannot face things without drink. This is a time of emotional panic and the patient has fearful visions of going down-hill to ruin "like Uncle Henry," or his father "who drank himself to death," or some acquaintance who "finished up in an asylum."

We know that emotion sensitizes the brain to hypnosis and that when emotion enters the picture reason is relegated to the background. An idea introduced in this condition has all the force of a strong hypnotic suggestion. Can we regard alcoholism as the result of a posthypnotic suggestion self-given in an accidentally self-induced hypnotic state?

Certainly the behavior of the alcoholic would seem to support the theory. Few alcoholics *like* alcohol but feel *compelled* to take it against their better judgment, in much the same way as a deeply hypnotized person will later, in the waking state, feel *compelled* to carry out some foolish posthypnotic suggestion.

Another point in favor is that alcoholics are *usually very susceptible* and make good hypnotic subjects so that the possibility of their having hypnotized themselves is very likely.

It should be noted that contrary to popular belief it is not necessary to "fall asleep," "close the eyes," or be "stretched out and sat upon," as in stage shows, to be hypnotized. Even in such shows during exhibitions of "mass hypnosis," dozens of people in the audience in full waking state will be found who are unable to "unlock" their clasped hands until permitted to do so by the hypnotist.

Finally there is the undisputed fact that hypnosis *when properly used* can and does cure cases of long standing alcoholism. It is a fundamental law that what can be caused by suggestion can be cured by suggestion and, even in all the orthodox treatments, there is a big element of suggestion. In treating alcoholism by hypnosis it is not sufficient or desirable to employ the usual naïve stage or amateur technique by simply saying, "Now you cannot drink," "Drink will make you sick," etc. Treatment should be aimed at enabling the patient not only to give up alcohol but teaching him how to face life and its problems in an adult fashion so that there can be no relapse. With proper planning this can be done in a relatively short space of time and using only a light to medium form of hypnosis which practically anybody can achieve. Usually a preliminary session to discuss the case and explain the nature of the treatment, followed by half-a-dozen sessions of hypnosis, is sufficient to establish a cure.

Treatment by hypnosis has the advantage that there is no stigma attached to it as with institutional treatment and patients can continue at their occupations and live an ordinary life. One condition is essential—*the patient must really want to get well*. The man who applies for treatment because he fears going down to ruin and desperately wants to give up drinking can be easily cured. The man who is dragged along by his wife to be cured, and who secretly has no desire to be cured, is unlikely to respond very easily if at all. Fortunately such cases are few and far between and the majority of victims are only too anxious to cooperate.

The following cases will give some idea of the value of hypnosis in the treatment of alcoholism:

CASE 1. Medical man, 45. The patient had been in the habit of taking excessive alcohol over a period of years. He had started drinking in the usual way, first of all on social occasions, then increasing gradually to ease the strain of general practice until he realized suddenly that he could not face life without it. If unable to get ordinary alcoholic drinks he would even drink methylated spirits. Various treatments had been tried without success and the patient was rapidly going downhill. Five sessions of hypnosis at weekly intervals were sufficient to remove the craving entirely. There has been no relapse over a considerable period of time and his wife reports that he is mentally, morally and physically a different man. His doctor wrote . . . "I am very interested in Dr. . . . . because he was cured by hypnotism while actually drinking and when institutional and other treatment had entirely failed."

CASE 2. Mrs. . . . . 50. This patient had had a very hard and tragic life. She had started drinking socially but increased the dose and frequency to ease the shock of losing her first husband. When her second husband was killed and she lost her only daughter in tragic circumstances she took more and more alcohol to drown her sorrow. Eventually she realized with a shock that she could not do without it and had fearful visions of what her end would be as "there was drink in the family." When seen she was drinking a bottle of whisky a day and all other treatment had failed. A few sessions of hypnosis were sufficient to establish a complete cure and there has been no relapse over a long period in spite of trying conditions.

CASE 3. Married man, 40. The patient had started drinking during service abroad, merely as a social habit. This increased to ease general worries and responsibilities in later life. Realization that he relied on alcohol so much came as a great shock to him as he had "seen what it had done to others." When seen, the patient was drinking heavily and trying to forget. A few sessions removed all desire for drink and over a year later his doctor wrote to say . . . "he has been quite free of any tendency to alcoholism since he had hypnotic treatment."

CASE 4. Mrs. . . . . 50. This patient had been introduced to alcohol in her school days abroad where, apparently, on special feast days the whole school received enough to make them merry! She continued drinking socially but increased the dose considerably when she lost her husband. After a time the patient suddenly realized with a shock how much she depended upon alcohol. She became afraid of her future as "there was drink in the family." When seen she was drinking very heavily—was never really sober in fact—and even took bottles of drink to bed with her. Again a few sessions of hypnotic suggestion were sufficient to abolish the craving completely.

CASE 5. Mrs. . . . . 45. This patient began drinking for social reasons. As her social duties increased, involving personal appearances under rather trying conditions, she drank more and more to cover up her nervousness. She realized suddenly with a shock how much she relied upon alcohol and had visions of "finishing up in an asylum like her father." From then on she drank more and more, endeavoring to drown this and other fears. All orthodox treatment had been unable to help, but she responded perfectly to a few sessions of hypnosis.

CASE 6. Mr. . . . . married man, 45. This case is especially interesting because it is generally believed that an alcoholic cannot drink socially but must give up alcohol of all kinds completely if he wants to be cured. This patient had started drinking to be "one of the crowd" but increased the dose to enable him to face business worries. There was a history of alcoholism in the family and the patient suddenly conceived a great fear of going downhill. This caused him to drink more than ever. The patient insisted, against advice, that he must be allowed to drink beer in moderation "for business reasons," but begged to be freed from the curse of alcohol in the form of spirits to which he was addicted. He was warned that it was generally considered impossible for an alcoholic to do this. However, as he insisted, he was treated with hypnosis and reported himself free from any desire for spirits. A year later his wife wrote to say . . . "he has been quite all right since having hypnotic treatment and is wonderfully changed. He is now able to manage a new business. He still drinks beer but that is all and that is in fact a stern test indeed. I know this to be true because I could always tell immediately when he had been drinking spirits or wines and now I am confident of his cure."

Although not generally advised, this case and others like it show that it is *possible* for a former alcoholic to drink sociably. Hypnotism is not a "cure all" and will almost certainly fail in cases which have no *real* desire to be cured. A typical case was that of Mr. . . . . who was forced to apply for treatment (very reluctantly) by his wife. As she had told him she would leave him if he did not stop drinking, and as this was the one thing he desired, then it was not surprising that cooperation was nil and hypnosis failed!

These typically successful cases, however, and many others like them show that there is a very real place for hypnosis in the treatment of alcoholism.

HYPNOTIC CONTROL
OF MENSTRUAL PAIN

BY

WILLIAM S. KROGER, M.D.

AND

S. CHARLES FREED, M.D.

————————

The treatment of functional dysmenorrhea is still in a relatively unsatisfactory stage. Considerable effort has been expended in obtaining results not only with analgesics and sedatives but also with expensive endocrine preparations. None has proved exceptionally successful, but a wide variety of these preparations have been reported to yield relief in some patients.

It is acknowledged by many investigators that the relief from painful menstruation may often be the result of unintended suggestion derived from the therapy, regardless of what preparations are used. Such results are in agreement with the theory held by many, that there is a definite psychic factor associated with functional dysmenorrhea, and the principal feature of this is a lowered threshold to pain. Thus, contractions of the uterus are conveyed to the consciousness of the individual, whereas normally these contractions are not registered as pain. In some patients this lowered threshold to pain may be due to an underlying psychosomatic condition.

Since relatively weak suggestion has been partially effective in bringing relief, a type of psychotherapy, combining the use of more effective suggestion as the main implement, would seem desirable for treating this condition. Such a mechanism where powerful suggestion can be transmitted is available in the form of hypnosis.

Certain functional disorders, especially in gynecology and obstetrics, lend themselves remarkably well to this form of therapy and should command the attention of the clinician. Because many of the successful results in treating functional dysmenorrhea are on the basis of suggestion, we have selected this condition for the possibility of demonstrating relief through hypnotism, by means of which powerful and concentrated suggestion may be easily applied. We wish to emphasize that hypnosis is only a means toward treatment, and when combined with modern psychoanalytical skill and knowledge it can be a much more effective treatment of functional dysmenorrhea than any of the methods in use today.

CASES TREATED BY HYPNOSIS AND POSTHYPNOTIC SUGGESTION

The following procedure was used in four cases: after rapport is established with the patient, hypnosis is induced.

Suggestions are made in this state that the next menses may be free from pain or without excessive discomfort. Also suggestions are made that the next menses will be normal in all respects. Posthypnotic suggestions last about a month, and when repeated the desired effect may become permanent. All four cases were permanently cured using this method. Only one treatment was necessary to bring permanent relief in two cases. Three to twelve treatments were necessary for the other two cases.

The following case histories are typical of the methods and results.

CASE 1. Miss L. S., aged 17, had painful menses since the age of nine and a half. The menses were always irregular. She was forced to retire to bed for 24 to 36 hours after the onset of the pain which usually occurred about 12 hours after the period began. It consisted of acute lower abdominal cramps accompanied by considerable nervousness, nausea and tension. She had received extensive therapy including dilatation and curettage, analgesics and endocrine preparations. A presacral sympathectomy was being considered, to which she had agreed.

On August 2, 1941, deep hypnosis was easily induced. Suggestions were given to the effect that her next menses would be free from discomfort; that every night before going to sleep she would say to herself, "I will have no pain. I have no dread and anticipation for my next period." These suggestions under hypnosis were repeated seven times between August 2, 1941, and August 29, 1941, The period began on September 6, 1941, and was remarkably free from pain although there were slight cramps. She did not have to go to bed. After four hypnotic treatments at weekly intervals, using the same suggestions, her next menses on October 11, was entirely normal in every respect. For one year, without any further treatments, she has been free from pain, nervousness and all menstrual discomfort. In addition her periods have been regular.

CASE 2. Miss D. K., aged 19, had severe dysmenorrhea of three years' duration. It consisted of severe lower abdominal cramps accompanied by depression. The menses usually lasted for four days during which time she was unable to work.

The patient had consulted several physicians and had tried all kinds of hypodermic treatments and drugs with little or no results. On November 15, 1941, deep hypnosis was induced easily. The same suggestions were given as in Case 1. The patient was hypnotized at weekly intervals twice before her next period. On December 6, the menses were entirely normal. All menstrual periods have been normal since that time. She has been relieved of her depression entirely and can now even practice acrobatic dancing during her entire menstrual period.

CASES TREATED BY HYPNOANALYSIS AND AGE REGRESSION

It occurred to us that some cases of functional dysmenorrhea present a characteristic constitutional psychosomatic pattern which may be responsible for a lowered pain threshold. Because latent psychogenic factors contribute to the intensity and production of the dysmenorrhea, they must be determined by an exhaustive study of the personality. We have utilized age regression with hypnoanalysis, which is a rapid form of psychoanalysis under hypnosis, in five cases. The patient is regressed to a pre-adolescent age or reverted to the age prior to the onset of the dysmenorrhea. The patient is then slowly reoriented to the present chronological age. The development of emotional conflicts, personality changes, inhibitions or harmful habit patterns can be discovered. Appropriate suggestions are then made toward their removal. After the patient's consciousness is reeducated by intensive psychotherapy under hypnosis, a cure may be effected readily. A total amnesia for the entire menstrual period may be produced in some individuals.

However, it must be emphasized that hypnosis when used in these cases is only the means toward treatment, not the cure itself. It effectively speeds up the entire analytical process. The use of hypnoanalysis and age regression readily extracts intimate facts held in the subconscious mind which ordinarily would not be available to the physician with the patient in the wakened state.

Five patients were regressed using this method. Two patients had never experienced orgasms. One patient, whose case is described below, had no improvement because of the husband's sexual impotence and premature ejaculation. However, the husband in spite of treatment never was able to have satisfactory intercourse with his wife. The other patient had complete relief from menstrual discomfort after attaining orgasms following suitable conditioning while in the hypnotic state. Her husband was normal sexually. One patient was a habitual masturbator who had complete recovery after adequate sexual advice was given. One had dysmenorrhea only during two unhappy marriages and between these marriages she had no dysmenorrhea. This patient was only partially improved since she is still unhappily married to her second husband. One woman had dysmenorrhea only after excessive sexual excitement without intercourse. Marriage was advised in this case. Shortly after the patient followed our advice and married, the painful periods ceased.

The following case histories are typical of the methods and results.

CASE 1. Mrs. R. B., aged 31, married eleven years. Severe dysmenorrhea began immediately after marriage. Cramps preceded onset of flow and became more severe as bleeding ensued accompanied by headache and nervousness. She was hypnotized easily on March 6. Suggestions were given at weekly intervals as in the cases previously described. The next menses on April 2, was unimproved. Four applications of hypnosis at weekly intervals were made prior to onset of period on May 1, with only slight improvement. On May 7, she was regressed to the age of 18 and gradually reoriented to the present age. The following facts were elicited. She had never had an orgasm while married even though her husband was potent sexually. She abhorred coitus and considered it "something to be endured." Following the birth of her second child three years ago her libido was lost completely. Her husband threatened a divorce. The patient professes some love for her husband and a desire to at least satisfy him. One week later under hypnosis, suggestions were given to the effect that she would have an orgasm the next time she had intercourse. Since she had experienced orgasms before her marriage there was no need to describe the subjective sensations. These suggestions were repeated at three weekly intervals during which time she abstained from intercourse. Coitus occurred on June 10, and although not accompanied by an orgasm the patient stated "she almost felt one." Her husband was told to have intercourse on June 14, and he was given proper sexual advice. This advice was followed and the patient experienced an orgasm. Her sexual life has been satisfactory since then and all menstrual discomfort disappeared completely.

CASE 2. Mrs. L. F., aged 20, had painful periods for the past two years. Extreme nervousness was present during the entire period. For the past year her menses have been most irregular. Patient states, "she began to have menstrual cramps at the age of 18." All therapy was of no avail. Pain began on the first day and was present on the second and fifth days. She was hypnotized on October 4, and was regressed to the age of 17 where the following facts were elicited. Her menses first became painful after meeting her husband whom she never loved. She had never achieved an orgasm with her husband during intercourse although this occurred during preliminary love-making. Her husband was inadequate sexually. She was given posthypnotic suggestions to the effect that she would have an orgasm during intercourse and her menses would be painless. On October 11, the suggestions under hypnosis were repeated. On October 17, the menses were free from discomfort until the fifth day. Orgasms were not achieved. The next menses was on December 7, and was painful and the patient failed to return for further treatment.

DISCUSSION

In this small series of nine cases treated as described above, the results are most gratifying. All the patients were referred by competent gynecologists. No obvious cause for the cyclic pain could be demonstrated in any of the cases. Various therapeutic procedures had been tried on each patient with disappointing results.

The inconvenience of using hypnosis is relatively negligible when compared with symptomatic therapy and the expense of multiple injections required for much of the endocrine treatment. The technique described here can easily be acquired by any physician. In addition, temporary dysfunction of the ovaries is not induced and the cures are relatively complete and permanent.

This form of psychotherapy, which acts by raising the pain threshold directly or through the eliciting of psychogenic factors indirectly causing the pain, is a convenient and effective therapeutic procedure for permanently curing this ordinarily refractory condition.

HYPNOTHERAPY FOR CHILDREN

BY

DR. GORDON AMBROSE

It is almost 50 years since an account of any importance has been written in relation to child psychiatry and treatment by hypnotherapy. Pioneer contributions were made in England by Bramwell, in France by Voisin, Berillon and Liebeault and in Germany by Bauer and Teuscher. Liebeault (1883) prepared a review showing the susceptibility of children to hypnosis and Beaunis stressed, in a later table, the ease of inducing a deep trance in children. Berillon found children curiously suggestible, and in 250 cases hypnotized 80 percent at the first attempt. In view of the earlier writers' emphasis of cures in all the functional conditions of childhood, it is surprising that more use has not been made of a therapy both rapid and successful. The ease of hypnotizing children has recently been stressed by Vernon Braithwaite (1950), Kanner (1948) and Ambrose (1950). The tendency has so far been for child guidance clinics to treat cases of anxiety and the like in children, by systematic psychotherapy, playtherapy or psychoanalysis, all time-consuming and necessarily limited to few patients. Treatment of these cases by hypnotherapy offers an alternative method, having the great advantage of taking up much less time and so allowing for the treatment of many more patients.

It is universally recognized that anxiety in children is by far the commonest symptom of emotional disturbance and that the anxiety is fundamentally a state of tension, in which the small mind is overloaded with energy. In adults the very fact of a discussion with a good listener may result in some relief of this pent-up tension, and in children the same result might be expected. However, children tend to be extremely reticent in describing unpleasant experiences and indeed the small mind has great difficulty in wording and explaining anxiety, which is so often not even at conscious level. It has not been sufficiently stressed that suggestions, given while the child is relaxed and sleepy, have a striking effect on this mounting tension, causing an almost instantaneous lessening of the tension, with subsequent relief of the associated anxiety and a greater feeling of security, so obviously lacking in the anxious child. The results obtained by the technique are so striking that it is considered worth while to write this communication.

The results of hypnotic treatment in 50 cases may be classified as follows: in 30 cases the therapy resulted in the cure of symptoms and over the past three years no relapses have been recorded. In the remaining 20 cases, 15 of the children were relieved and five showed little change. It must be stressed that in all 50 cases the striking result of the therapy was an immediate lessening of tension, a factor of immense and immeasurable importance in these tension-anxiety symptoms, and thus an admittance by the child of "I don't seem to worry about it any more."

It will be seen in the later review of some of the cases that six children had been treated by ordinary psychological methods, i.e., systematic psychotherapy, playtherapy, suggestion and in one case by psychoanalysis, over a considerable time, without any very obvious slackening of the fundamental symptomatology. However, after the use of hypnotherapy there appeared a rapid and startling change in the pathology of the child's symptoms and general outlook, which was discernable to the doctor and parents.

The present results give an approximate impression only. After a longer follow-up period it is hoped to publish a more detailed analysis which would necessarily take into account such obviously important factors as the environmental background of the children treated, the parents' reaction to psychological probing, and the nature and duration of previous treatment.

SELECTION OF CASES

Many children seen in a child guidance clinic, although presenting obvious psychological difficulties, are not necessarily suitable for hypnotherapy. Ordinary superficial psychotherapy practiced by the general practitioner or psychiatrist would be adequate, and others would be cured by specialized forms of psychological therapy.

Children are selected as suitable for hypnotherapy under the following criteria: (1) The degree and depth of the psychological trauma present and the attitude of the parents to this reaction, (2) Duration and degree of tension shown by the child, (3) Where other methods of psychotherapy have failed or have made no very rapid strides, (4) Patients should preferably not be under the age of 6.

TECHNIQUE

Few of the earlier writers discuss a different technique, in adults or children, for the induction of hypnosis. Modern views maintain hypnosis is primarily a function of the interpersonal relationship existing between the subject and the hypnotist. Whereas in the adult the technique for the induction of hypnosis might depend on how far the hypnotist can adapt his technique to satisfy the personality needs of his subject, it will be readily appreciated that children have a personality easier satisfied and accept the hypnotist with adequate cooperation.

It cannot be too strongly stressed that for purposes of achieving therapeutic results quickly and with the least amount of difficulty, it is not necessary to obtain deep hypnosis. It will also be appreciated that in child psychiatry where the main importance is undoubtedly a happy parent-child relationship, and where psychotherapy is aimed at this relationship and all that it stands for, any technique that enables the physician to produce a positive transference with the child, quickly and successfully, is of inestimable value.

It will be found in practice that children are adept at achieving a light trance and the technique required to hypnotize them is minimal. The three cardinal rules are (a) gain the child's confidence, (b) tell him what you are going to do, (c) use any technique.

The child is told to close his eyes and relax; a preliminary discussion on how to make the muscles loose is very easily understood by the youngest of children and takes only a few minutes. Suggestions are given—"Your eyes are heavy, all your muscles are loose, you are very tired and drowsy, tired and drowsy, you are very sleepy, you sleep," and these suggestions are repeated. When enough relaxation has been achieved, curative suggestions are proceeded with. These curative suggestions take the form of reassurance and naturally will be based on a preliminary discussion with parents and child, when the psychiatrist will be enabled to grasp the salient facts that allow him to decide the type and severity of the case, the probable prognosis, the methods of psychotherapy suitable to the case, and an appraisal of the chances of rapport with the parents, possibly the most fundamental task in child guidance work.

In the past the difficulty of using this technique has been the implications attached to the word "hypnosis." The general public and, even more so, the medical profession, are oddly critical of hypnotic procedure and indeed the majority of individuals have no clear idea of what constitutes hypnosis. Today, with the word appearing on almost every page of the national press, in behooves the profession to educate the public, if and when they require knowledge on this subject, a difficult procedure when the medical profession is largely ignorant of this recognized technique in psychotherapy, and would allow their scientific minds to be clogged with superstitions handed down to them since the days of Mesmer. There would be no problem if the individual remembers that, at some time or another, each and every child has been subjected to hypnosis or at least, a modified form of hypnosis. Every mother and nurse uses the technique in order to ensure sleep for their infant— the crooning of a song, the telling of a bedtime story, the soothing words of reassurance, are simply the arts of the hypnotist and serve precisely the same purpose—a method of relaxation during which it is possible to influence a child by suggestion and reeducation.

Children vary in their immediate response to hypnotherapy. The majority, obviously perturbed, anxious and unhappy when seen, seemingly lose these symptoms of tension rapidly and effectively at the first session of hypnotherapy. At least six sessions are necessary to ensure permanent relief from symptoms; these sessions, at weekly intervals, follow a set routine, each case is allotted 30 minutes, 20 minutes for discussion with parents and the remaining 10 minutes for hypnotherapy with the child—it will be appreciated that the extra time given to the parents is for their reeducation, a more painstaking and longer process than is generally necessary with the child. It will be found in practice that psychotherapy to the parents, hypnotherapy to the child, achieves results so much quicker and more permanent than other more tedious methods of child guidance.

CASE 1. A male child aged 6½ was seen by me with a history of asthma attacks since birth. The attacks were typically periodic and were characterized by severe and slight attacks. The severe attacks occurred about once monthly and the slight attacks every two–three days. He also complained of attacks of irritation of the skin of the face, and backs of his legs, the asthma alternated with the eczema. The skin rash necessitated gloves to prevent scratching at night. The bad attacks of asthma were associated with bronchitis and pyrexia was severe enough to warrant treatment with sulpha-chemotherapy on several occasions. The asthma was controlled by ephedrine given through an atomizer, previously injections of adrenaline had been given by the practitioner in charge of the case, but ceased after July, 1948; all the new and most of the old treatments had been tried with varying success.

The boy's mother was seemingly overanxious and excessively interested in the asthma, she had never been told that reassurance by herself would help the boy to overcome the attacks. The maternal grandmother, living in the same house, was a chronic sufferer from asthma for over 50 years. There seemed to be a relationship between the two asthmas, frequently attacks would appear at the same time. The boy's father had been killed in the last war and the mother married again, the second husband had legally adopted the child and was a good father to the boy.

The boy was intelligent, cooperative and anxious to get well. The mother proved equally intelligent and cooperative, and after three sessions had an excellent insight into her child's illness and the factors aggravating the condition. The child was seen once weekly for six weeks. On the third visit he was in an acute attack of asthma but insisted on getting out of bed and visiting me, explaining to his mother that if he could get to see me the asthma would never come back. On the fifth visit he wanted to know why he had to see me still and again insisted, "Why do I have to go when I'm well now?" His words proved prophetic for he has not suffered an attack of any description, asthma or eczema, for over one year.

The case is interesting for several reasons. The attacks had dated from birth and, together with the infantile eczema, showed a well marked "allergic syndrome." The grandmother's attacks, undoubtedly "psychological" in origin (they first appeared at the age of 22), acted as more fuel for the fire, and indeed her attitude to the boy's illness, and my treatment, was a difficult one to overcome; she claimed that psychological treatment for asthma was "stuff and nonsense, and indicative of the years we live in." Nevertheless she did cooperate after seeing the improvement early in the treatment. The mother was surprised and horrified that she would have to ignore the attacks, and allow the child to play with other children if he looked as though he was in for an attack. At the third session, when the child appeared in an attack, this was aborted by suggestion during hypnotherapy.

CASE 2. A child aged 12 was brought to the Department of Psychiatry by his parents because it was noticed that for three years he was overshy, bullied by smaller and younger children, could not concentrate at school and had nightmares and insomnia. His parents stated that he would give away anything and everything if threats were made to him. He was easily reduced to tears, but at home was given to aggressive outbursts and temper tantrums, and the parents could do nothing with the boy. It transpired that a traumatic episode at the age of 9 had been responsible for these symptoms, the boy had been attacked by a man and had been forced to masturbate him under threats. Before this incident he had been happy and bright and easily managed at school. Great excitement had attended this unhappy episode, and the police had been informed, leading to a court sequel. The parents had not felt the necessity to explain things to the child and "didn't know much about sexual matters anyway." Reassurance and explanations, which the child thoroughly understood, produced a certain improvement, but the boy was obviously unhappy, and it was decided to use hypnotherapy. He was seen at three sessions of ten minutes each session and there was an immediate improvement. He showed more courage, the nightmares ceased, he became better tempered and markedly less aggressive at home, did better at school and has remained so for over three years.

This case illustrates a too common occurrence in young children frightened by sexual perverts. The unknown presents a problem which the child turns over and over in his mind, and as the solution eludes him anxiety supervenes. The initial trauma was naturally aggravated by the panic reactions of the adults, at the time of the crime, and the eventual court proceedings, without adequate explanations to the child. A certain amount of "abreaction" was accomplished by the use of hypnosis in this case, which resulted in an easing of symptoms by a lessening of tension.

CASE 3. A female child of 10 was brought by her mother because she had suddenly shown a violent fear of darkness, refused to cross the road on her own, would not sleep by herself, and became almost unmanageable at home. Her father had been desperately ill for years and, before dying, was quite blind and in constant pain; the children had to be quiet during the day, and were answerable to their mother for everything. The mother was markedly unstable before the long illness of her husband, having shown hysterical symptoms on occasions. The child, however, was captain of her form, and a prefect at school, and was a first-class little sportswoman. Directly the father died the child showed these acute anxiety symptoms. The same procedure was adopted in this case as in Case 2, i.e., systematic psychotherapy over four weeks, to both child and parent, produced a certain improvement, but the child was still afraid of the dark, and seemed unhappy, and the obvious fear and tension required something stronger than conscious suggestion. The exact reassurances given to her in the waking state, and actually taken down at the time of the sessions when first seen, were given to her during the first hypnotic session. The result was astonishing. She slept on her own, smiled when she was asked if she feared the dark and became, almost overnight, a confident, happy little schoolgirl.

CASE 4.   A girl of 11 was brought by her mother with a history of blinking of the eyes and fidgeting since the age of 5. The child was difficult to manage, aggressive and seemingly full of anxiety. The mother stated that her daughter appeared frustrated and was given to tantrums at the least provocation, she admitted that her own nerves were not so good, she had recently obtained a divorce from her husband, she had not been living with him for years (the child had never known her father), and was obviously tense and anxious herself.

When the child was first seen there were gross tics present. The blinking of the eyes was incessant and accompanied by expiratory "grunts," as her breath was forcibly expelled; the involuntary grunts occurred about six times a minute. The first session was amusing; suggestions that the child was relaxed and sleepy sounded odd as the grunts became more aggravated. Notwithstanding, however, and although only the slightest relaxation was obtained, a week later there was obvious improvement in the movements. Later she obtained a medium degree of relaxation. The mother, when first seen, displayed very little insight into her daughter's difficulties—she was rigorous in her outlook and had been projecting her own conflicts and repressions to her child. Although antagonistic and frankly skeptical at the first few sessions, by the sixth she had attained excellent insight, and was cooperative and eager to help her daughter. The anxiety part of the case had cleared. However, the tics persisted, but in a modified form, the grunts had disappeared and the blinking was very much less. Later reports of the child confirmed that she is happy at school and shows slight blinking of the eyelids, especially when tired or upset.

Like many symptoms which are not associated with serious bodily ill health, tics have received somewhat superficial treatment in medical teaching. Authorities stress several factors in their aetiology, overstrain at school, lack of occupation, illness and fright being a few of them. The value of the technique in this case was the achieving of an immediate lessening of tension in the child. The symptoms were thus improved and the psychiatrist was enabled to achieve a quicker and more satisfactory rapport with the parent—a vital matter in a case of this description.

CASE 5.   A boy aged 13 was brought to me because he was slacking at school, seemed to be full of anxiety, and had wet his bed almost every night since a baby. His mother was a brilliant scholar, a university graduate and lecturer before her marriage. She married her first cousin. She is the boy's driving force, the father placid and easygoing. The boy himself stated that he was sick of worrying over his bed-wetting. He found it increasingly difficult to get his homework done, and had recently lost interest in his music (he showed promise at the piano). He was unable to concentrate, and found everything difficult. He had a long journey to school (he won a scholarship) and his parents were seriously thinking of changing the school to one nearer his home. It was very obvious that the mother showed gross interest and anxiety over the boy's bladder.

His intelligence tests showed an I.Q. between 120 and 125, and he scored 54 out of 60 in his Matrix (Raven) test. Hypnotherapy was commenced rather tardily in this case due to a surgical condition (spina bifida). However, after the first session the boy showed a marked improvement in his anxiety symptomatology. The first thing he told me was that he had no worry, he felt confident that he would stop wetting, and that "even if I don't I won't worry." He went to a camp and had five dry nights and two wet ones. The improvement ceased immediately he returned home, but the anxiety and slacking at school got rapidly better. He became top of his form, from nearly bottom, and passed a higher examination in pianoforte. The wetting persists but he insists he no longer worries about it as he did.

This case illustrates Moodie's conception of nocturnal enuresis. Moodie considers that enuresis arises in many cases from a disorder of organic function and the extra tension which is represented by anxiety accentuates the condition, so that symptoms develop. This boy was deeply hypnotized on several occasions and was a somnambule. While receiving suggestions he remained dry, thus supporting Braithwaite's contention that nocturnal enuresis cannot be a psychogenic illness, as hypnosis often fails to cure the condition.

CASE 6.   A girl of 18 years was seen by me and gave a history of fits since the age of 14. She was first seen at the King's College

Hospital in 1943, and a diagnosis of idiopathic epilepsy was made. She had been given tablets of phenobarbitone, which did not adequately control the fits. Later epanutin tablets in a dose of 0.2G first thing in the morning, 0.1G midday and 0.1G at night, together with phenobarbitone (luminal) ½ gr. three times daily, adequately controlled the fits. She had forgotten to take the midday dose of epanutin (sodium diphenyl hydantoinate) on several occasions and suffered a fit each time she forgot.

She was first seen by me on January 27th, 1951. The only significant factor elicited from her was that at the age of 8 she was interfered with by a man, while taking her baby brother for a walk in a park. There was a great commotion and she was brought home in a police car. Just before her periods she feels tense and anxious and many of the grand mal attacks have corresponded to the commencement of this cycle. She had over sixty grand mal attacks before seeing me.

At the first session she appeared sleepy and disinterested and it seemed that she was showing signs of mental deterioration. She was easily and deeply hypnotized and when seen seven days later appeared more alert and interested. On the 2nd of February she again forgot to take her midday dose of epanutin and suffered a grand mal attack at work, the same afternoon. She saw me on the 11th of February and told me that she would have to leave her employment, because of her illness. She appeared depressed and retarded and admitted that "life was hopeless and she would never get another job." Again seen on the 17th of February she was much brighter, she had been offered work as a cashier, a job she felt she could do adequately. After this session it was decided to stop the phenobarbitone tablets gradually.

She has been seen by me regularly once every 14 days. She is now taking epanutin 0.1G three times daily. She is alert, happy and confident that eventually the drug will be stopped altogether. She has not suffered a fit since 17th of February.

Many of the older writers have described the treatment and relief of this condition by hypnotherapy. Thus Bramwell, Voisin, Wood, Wetterstrand, de Jong and many others describe cases of epilepsy relieved and sometimes cured by hypnosis. There appears evidence that hypnotherapy controls the number of fits in this condition, and enables the patient to dispense with large doses of sedatives—the patient can be made more alert and confident and combined with adequate doses of epanutin, the number of fits are minimal, thus preventing deterioration, the great hazard in these unfortunate cases.

CASE 7. A boy of 14 was brought by his mother with the following history. After listening to a play on the wireless he showed peculiar behavior. He started to walk in his sleep, called out at night, said that men were following him. He was timid and frightened and easily reduced to tears. The whole picture was complicated by the history of an accident—several days before he had run his bicycle into the back of a lorry, while apparently daydreaming. It transpired, after further history taking, that the child had been seen at the Maudsley Hospital as an out-patient, and that he had a cousin who was a "bit queer." His parents were desperate, both suffering from lack of sleep, and told me that "they would have a nervous breakdown if something wasn't done." Hypnotherapy was commenced and he showed immediate improvement, especially in the more hysterical aspects of his case. He was seen the usual six times and recently a check-up showed that he had maintained his improvement. Naturally he remains a somewhat schizoid type, shut-in and somewhat shallow, but he has developed more courage, his nightmares have ceased, he is doing well at school and doesn't mind "boxing with the other boys."

In 1889 Berillon had written "When, however, children are . . . afflicted with infirmities, we ought to try to cure them by hypnotism, especially when their parents are in despair, owing to the failure of all other forms of treatment." This case amply illustrates these sentiments. The child had received treatment without apparent benefit and the parents were in despair, two reasons for a therapy capable of rapidly easing the tension in this previously unhappy child.

CASE 8. A boy of 14 was stated by his parents and teachers to be antagonistic to discipline, was stealing from other children at school and was a member of a gang roaming the streets at night, throwing stones, molesting adults and other children. Matrix and Binet-Simon tests showed an I.Q. of over 110. His father was inadequate, his mother full of "don'ts." The boy told me that he was constantly criticized by his two aunts, who were living in the same house; they appeared to expect too high a standard from him. He showed definite signs of psychopathy in his personality, thus he was excitable, impulsive, antisocial and aggressive. He told me that he could not tolerate people shouting at him and indeed on one occasion had shown a typical psychopathic reaction when shouted at by his employer. The boy was given a course of hypnotherapy over six weeks and showed a startling change in his behavior. He became thoughtful, hard-working and friendly, gave up his gang, and showed a definite personality change.

The parents of this child were never seen. He was brought to me by his employer, and his father died while he was receiving treatment. The reason that this child has not relapsed is due to the employer, who has ensured a satisfactory environment, and has taken a personal interest in the case. The boy has remained well for four years. Hypnotherapy in early cases of delinquency offers a quicker and more certain method of treating the intelligent juvenile delinquent.

DISCUSSION

The foregoing cases show, in several children, the result of frustration, conflict and repression. The child is unable to achieve a stable background and happiness, the birthright of every child is destroyed.

It has been increasingly obvious to me that, in certain cases, children, even when reassured by the psychiatrist, aided and abetted by the parents, have failed to achieve a release of tension; this pent-up emotion continues in spite of psychotherapy to parents and child. Hypnotherapy offers them an immediate release from this tension. A practical consideration is that treatment can be carried out in the out-patient department, and a limited number of consultations are required compared with systematic psychotherapy and analytical methods. Most impressive is the rapidity of the result from this form of treatment and the infrequency of relapse. It will be seen from the cases described that, in general, great improvement was obtained after the second or third session and in all of 50 cases so treated improvement was obtained after the first session, sufficient for both parents and doctor to notice and remark upon. All the cases were cleared or improved.

Two of the cases illustrated were treated by systematic psychotherapy over an extended period, and it was shown that although there was apparent improvement, it required hypnotherapy to release rudiments of tension still present in each child. Six other cases were treated in a like manner, as being typical of anxiety-tension in children, and showed the same result.

During the past few years the production of abreaction by drugs or gases has taken a place in recognized psychiatric therapy, the object of this abreaction being simply the release of tension. Sargant and Slater, Palmer, Rogerson, and Shorvon have all described the importance of this release of tension in psychiatrical cases in the adult; fortunately, in the child, it is unnecessary to adopt these somewhat dangerous but effective techniques, and hypnotherapy adequately relieves the young mind of tension and allows anxiety to disperse itself.

Maladjustment to the realities of life, arising from childhood development and environment, is one of the main underlying factors in all the neuroses. Any therapy that allows the physician to assist the child in adaptation and adjustment to the rigors of ordinary citizenship should not be neglected. Hypnotherapy does precisely this and by achieving cure or relief the psychiatrist is enabled to unravel the emotional content of the parents and ensure that the family unit is peaceful, happy and hygienic.

HYPNOSIS IN OBSTETRICS

BY

MILTON ABRAMSON, M.D., Ph.D.

AND

WILLIAM T. HERON, Ph.D.

We are coming to realize more and more that a number of the difficulties and ills which human beings suffer are caused by their beliefs, traditions, and customs. For example, it is a belief that a woman should and will suffer great pain in childbirth. The girl hears this throughout the years and it has a great suggestive effect upon her. The result is that she will likely suffer pain at childbirth simply because she is conditioned to expect it. That childbirth pain is not necessary is indicated by the experience of women in some other parts of the world where this expectation of pain does not exist. Such women look upon childbirth as a natural function which is not expected to cause any more discomfort than any other physiological function of the body. In their experience, childbirth is quick and painless. Since the patient is conditioned to expect pain, the physician is forced to use methods to try to alleviate this pain.

Obstetricians have for many years been seeking a method of pain relief for the parturient woman. This search has led to the development of a multiplicity of techniques utilizing drugs of many kinds, orally, parenterally, and locally. All of these methods, with the exception of the use of local anesthesia, suffer from the same drawback and that is that they are not entirely safe for both the mother and baby. The obstetrician in his search for the ideal obstetrical analgesic and anesthetic has, however, overlooked what the authors feel is a very important consideration in the care of the pregnant and parturient woman, and that is her proper psychological preparation for her lying-in period. Agreeing that patients have been given the best of physical care and preparation for their labors, we must admit that due to a lack of time and frequently of desire, we have not been preparing our patients mentally for a physical experience that should be one of the high points in the life of any woman.

Following the publication in 1944 of Grantly Dick Read's book, "Childbirth Without Fear," there has been an increasing interest shown by a number of men in this technique of pain relief for the patient in labor. Thoms and Goodrich[1] recently, among others, have corroborated Read's work.

Inasmuch as Read's technique depends on the use of education, relaxation, and suggestion, and inasmuch as hypnosis also depends on relaxation and suggestion, it was felt that if the Read technique was carried a step further and a trance state induced, the results could be improved.

Hypnosis in medicine and surgery is, of course, not new. Many surgical procedures, both major and minor, have been performed with the use of hypnosis as the only anesthetic. The difficulty has always been that the lay person has felt that there is something mysterious about the procedure and as a result has been fearful about submitting himself to it. Today, hypnosis is an integral part of the psychological sciences and a great deal of investigation is now being carried on in this field.

In one of the earliest and most complete investigations done on the use of hypnosis in obstetrics in 1922, Schultze-Rhonhof[2] achieved a success of 89.5 percent in seventy-six cases. He states that the disadvantages of the procedure are mainly the time necessary to condition the patient for delivery and the presence of someone at the time of labor who has been trained in the technique of handling these patients. These two disadvantages, as he points out, can very easily be eliminated.

Kroger,[3, 4] in two articles written in 1943, described the use of hypnosis both in obstetrics and for the treatment of dysmenorrhea. He was enthusiastic in citing the advantages of the method and gave no contraindications to its use. Greenhill[5] in commenting on this paper stated, "It is unfortunate that most physicians consider hypnotism as charlatanism, because hypnosis is exceedingly useful in various fields of medicine—it should be used more extensively in obstetrics and gynecology."

Kroger,[6] in another paper titled, "The Treatment of Psychogenic Disorders by Hypnoanalysis," describes the use of hypnoanalysis, particularly for the common complaint of frigidity in women, with excellent success.

Wolberg,[7] in speaking of the use of hypnosis in dentistry, obstetrics, and surgery, states, "The anesthesia under hypnosis is profound and except for major surgical procedures is as effective as chemical anesthesia." He states further, "Obvious advantages are the ease of administration, the immediate removal of anesthesia when desired, and the absence of postoperative reactions to the anesthetic." In speaking of its use in obstetrics, Wolberg states, "Where the patient responds positively to these (hypnotic) suggestions, a total absence of pain results and postpartum discomfort is minimal."

LeCron and Bordeaux[8] also discuss the use of hypnosis in obstetrics and gynecology in their recent book, "Hypnotism Today."

Personal communications from a number of physicians have been variable in their reaction to the use of hypnosis in obstetrics, ranging from enthusiastic approval of the technique to a noncommittal acceptance of it as another possible method of analgesia.

The older literature is replete with descriptions of the use of hypnosis in a large variety of ailments both in general medicine and obstetrics and surgery, but to date there has been no objective attempt to evaluate it in its true perspective and from an unbiased point of view.

It appeared desirable, therefore, to make a more extended study using no selection of cases except that the patient be willing to cooperate in this experiment. This procedure would then give a better idea of what the physician may hope to accomplish by the use of this technique on the general run of patients. By using a fairly large number of subjects, we may also assess the advantages and disadvantages of hypnosis, and come to a conclusion concerning the practicality of the method.

MATERIAL

The subjects in this experiment were partly private and partly clinic patients. No attempt was made to start these patients on the training at any specified period of their pregnancy. Nor was any attempt made to hold constant the number of training periods given to the patient. Therefore, the training periods of approximately thirty minutes each ranged from two to as many as eight, with an average of four per patient. Some subjects were started as early as the second month of pregnancy and others as late as the eighth month. The average for the group was the seventh month.

In the training periods an attempt was made to get as deep a stage of hypnosis as possible. There are, of course, large individual differences in this respect from the few who do not go into the hypnotic condition at all to those who go into the deepest somnambulistic trance. There is no adequate objective method of determining the depth of hypnosis except to give the subject a series of tests involving the induction of catalepsy, anesthesia, hallucination, and amnesia. The giving of more than the very simplest of these tests is not desirable from the professional point of view because it is difficult for the subject to understand the relationship, for example, between having an hallucination and having a baby; therefore, the subject may feel that she is being made an experimental guinea pig to satisfy the curiosity of the physician, and some subjects tend to resent this. Further, unless time is taken in reassuring the patient, she may be frightened when she experiences some of the phenomena which can be produced in the hypnotic state; such a situation is obviously unfortunate from a psychological point of view. For such reasons, no systematic attempt was made to determine the depth of trance in our subjects. One or two were obviously not influenced at all. Others were apparently in the somnambulistic state. In doing an experiment of this kind, one is torn between the desire to have very careful controls and measurements, and the desire to make the situation as nearly as possible what the physician will meet in his everyday practice. We have allowed the latter desire to dominate our procedure in the present study. The phenomenon which we stressed most with all the patients was relaxation. This is a condition which can be quite easily induced in the hypnotic state, even in the lighter trance, and the relaxation is frequently much more complete than the subject can immediately accomplish otherwise.

The techniques of inducing the hypnotic trance and the conditioning process will not be discussed in this report as all of the methods that we have used have been adequately described in many previous publications. It is our feeling that any acceptable method of trance induction serves the purpose.

In this study we have been particularly concerned with objective indication of the effects of the training. If we were to rely solely on the subjective estimates by the patients we would have an almost 100 percent favorable response. The patients felt that the training made parturition easier for them. It is a little difficult to understand upon what basis a primipara [one in first childbirth] would make such a statement except possibly that she found her labor not so difficult as she expected it to be. Although these subjective reports have some value we would prefer to rest the case for the training on objective evidence. In order to do this, it was necessary for comparative purposes to have a group of patients who have not been trained. This group, called the control group, was obtained by pulling records at random from the hospital files. From the hospital records then certain data were secured for both the trained, called the experimental group, and the control group.

RESULTS

Our experimental and control groups were quite comparable except for the fact that there were 62 percent of primiparas in the experimental group and 48 percent in the control.

The average length of the first stage was two hours less for the experimental group. This is significant; a difference of that magnitude could be expected to occur by chance only three times in one hundred.

The variability of the first stage of labor for the experimental group was also less than for the controls.

It is generally stated that the labor of the primipara is, on the average, longer than that of the multipara. Since we had 14 percent more primiparas in our experimental group than in our control, it is likely that the difference of two hours was less than it would have been had the percentage of primiparas in the two been equal.

The training was more effective for the primipara than for the multipara. It reduced the time of the first stage for the former on the average of 3.23 hours and for the latter by 1.79 hours.

COMMENT

There is no doubt that spectacular results can be obtained in some patients by the use of hypnosis during parturition, but these cases are not representative of gravid women in general. The ability to go into a hypnotic state is complicated and involves many personality factors in the patient as well as skill on the part of the hypnotist. At the present time it is possible to put only about 20 percent of normal adult individuals into the deepest hypnotic condition. It is with such subjects that one is likely to get the most spectacular results.

But we do not have to seek only these outstanding cases in order to establish appreciable benefits from prenatal hypnotic training. A mean reduction of 20 percent in length of the first stage of labor with a minimum of drug is certainly to be desired and especially so when the patients subjectively feel that they have received much help.

SUMMARY AND CONCLUSIONS

Prenatal training in hypnosis can be of definite benefit to patients during parturition. It may give very significant relief from the discomfort of labor even in cases which do not show the spectacular results sometimes obtained, which are so fond to the heart of many of those who dabble with hypnosis. An average reduction of two hours in length of the first stage of labor with a minimum of drug would seem to be a result which is eminently desirable. It is this stage which is so monotonous and fatiguing to the patient. If this stage is prolonged, minutes seem like hours, especially if through undue tension and apprehension each contraction brings severe discomfort.

The great difficulty in the use of hypnosis is the time and effort which are required on the part of the physician to give the prenatal training. Another difficulty is that the hospital staff is not trained to deal with patients in the hypnotic state. If we can overcome the first difficulty by mass training, it should not be hard to train adequately nurses and other members of the hospital staff in the proper care of such patients.

If these two difficulties can be overcome, we believe that the method will be practicable and holds significant promise toward the relief of the discomforts of parturition, with no possible risk to the patient or her baby.

HYPNOSIS AND
SUGGESTION IN OBSTETRICS

**GEORGE NEWBOLD, M.R.C.S., D.R.C.O.G.,
M.M.S.A.**

Below are given the histories of three cases in which use was made of the power of suggestion to the subconscious mind so that the activity of the normal conscious levels and the concomitant highly developed critical faculties were temporarily suspended.

CASE REPORTS

CASE 1. The patient, a primigravida aged 21, was admitted to hospital as an emergency with a diagnosis of obstructed labor, having been in the second stage of labor for six hours after a first stage of about twenty-four hours. On examination rather painful uterine contractions were still present, although they were much less severe than they had been, the vertex was engaged but a large caput had formed, and there was excessive molding of the foetal head. The cause of the delay appeared to be a relative disproportion between the presenting part and the outlet, together with incomplete anterior rotation of the occiput. The head was fitting extremely tightly in the birth canal and seemed completely "stuck." A condition of light hypnosis was induced and the patient was instructed to relax, which

125

she did sufficiently well to enable the occiput to be rotated more to
the front and the forceps to be applied correctly. During delivery
of the baby the mother was able to cooperate and use her own
expulsive muscles while traction was being made. She later stated
that she had had no actual pain but that she felt "like another
person." Although the tissues of the perineum were very thick,
only a very small episiotomy was required. The placenta was expelled
naturally after 20 minutes, and the baby, which cried lustily, weighed
just over 10 lb.

CASE 2.   A primigravida aged 32 with a twin pregnancy was
admitted to hospital as a booked case, having regularly attended
the antenatal clinic. Her membranes ruptured two hours after labor
pains had started, and progress was very slow, as is often the case
with multiple pregnancies, so that towards the end of the third
day of labor she was much distressed and exhausted in spite of the
administration at intervals of pethidine hydrochloride in doses of
100 mg. each and other sedatives such as chloral hydrate and potas-
sium bromide. The cervix was then a little more than two-thirds
dilated but was very oedematous, and the patient constantly reiter-
ated her strong desire to bear down with each contraction. Doubt-
less this inability to relax properly during the first stage was partly
responsible for the oedema and slow dilatation of the cervix. In
spite of the presence of painful uterine contractions therapeutic suggestion was attempted, and after about fifteen minutes the patient
began to respond and became much quieter and more relaxed. A few
minutes later she was sleeping, although strong contractions were
still occurring. The suggestion of "No pain" was continued at intervals for another ten minutes or so, and she remained asleep for
some hours. When reexamined later, on awakening, her condition
was much improved, the cervix being nearly fully dilated and the
oedema having disappeared. She then stated that she felt much
refreshed and that all she could remember was a feeling of drowsiness associated with a sensation of being "far away—as if I were
floating in space." The rest of the labor progressed normally and
satisfactorily and both babies were born in good condition.

CASE 3.   A primigravida aged 24 was admitted to hospital owing to a prolonged first stage and an impending uterine inertia. She had been in labor for between two and three days and was becoming exhausted and depressed. On examination the cervix was nearly three-quarters dilated and the membranes were still intact. A light hypnotic sleep was then induced and the suggestion made that she would sleep until it was time to "push the baby out." She slept, although slightly restless now and then, for some hours, and soon after waking second-stage contractions began and labor then continued normally and uneventfully.

These three cases illustrate to some extent what can be achieved if the so-called "subconscious mind" can be utilized in aiding the removal of fear and tension and the promotion of relaxation both of mind and of body.

HYPNOSIS IN
GYNECOLOGIC DISORDERS

BY

WILLIAM S. KROGER, M.D.

A method which offers a relatively short and effective treatment when properly applied in functional gynecologic disorders is hypnoanalysis.

Hypnoanalysis has been used successfully to ameliorate many sensations of an unpleasant nature. It is known to be an effective and rapid form of therapy. Hypnoanalysis is a valuable adjunct to our therapeutic armamentarium because it effectively speeds up the diagnosis and obviates prolonged therapy.

Many investigators acknowledge that the relief of psychogynecic conditions results from unintentional suggestions, *irrespective of the therapy used.* Since weak suggestion has been effective in bringing about cures, a type of psychotherapy utilizing modern and scientific suggestion and analysis as the main implement should be much more effective.

Pure hypnosis as described by the earlier investigators, Forel, Bernheim, Liebault, and Charcot, has been found wanting in many respects because only symptoms were removed. Hypnoanalysis, a combination of hypnosis and psychoanalysis, is a rational psychotherapeutic procedure. It is more effective because "insight" into the basic emotional difficulties responsible for the symptoms are recognized by the patient as the mechanism of cure.

Hypnoanalysis elicits underlying psychogenic and behavior disorders and enables the therapist and patient to ascertain the factors responsible for the symptom complex. It is used as a means of penetrating below the resistances of the patient and is helpful in integrating, synthesizing, and enforcing new and more wholesome attitudes. Also new personality patterns can be engrafted. Most important of all, it speeds up an ordinarily slow process.

The following case histories are typical of our methods:

CASE 1. Mrs. P. E., aged 36 years. History of severe headaches since the age of ten, accompanied by photophobia, dizziness, nausea, and vomiting. Lower abdominal pain for sixteen years' duration. Palpitation, fatigue, nervousness, and suicidal tendencies, more marked during the past year.

Obstetric: Spontaneous delivery, 1932. Vaginal cesarean at $6\frac{1}{2}$ months. Pregnancy terminated because of the headaches.

Gynecologic: Menses: onset at age of 15 years, "first period frightened her to death," irregular, dysmenorrhea occurred immediately after marriage.

Complete medical, gynecologic, and neurological examinations were negative for organic pathology. An electroencephalogram was within normal limits.

Onset and Course—Patient states that her headaches began when she was 10 years old. Since then she consulted numerous physicians and clinics in America without obtaining relief. After a wide variety of symptomatic therapy, hypnosis was decided upon. The patient was hypnotized during a typical "migraine attack"; complete relief for the symptom was obtained. She was disassociated, and a specific amnesia produced for her true identity. The headaches always disappeared during the induction of this phenomenon of hypnosis. The patient tacitly acknowledged that the headaches, abdominal pain, and other symptoms might be on a neurotic basis, and hypnoanalysis was advised. The frigidity or symptom complex responsible for the above complaints was not mentioned at this time.

Hypnoanalytic therapy started with intensive training under hypnosis until the patient became a "somnambule."

In the somnambulistic stage the patient was easily reverted to earlier periods of life. The information elicited concerning her early life ordinarily would have taken a much longer period under psychoanalysis. During this process of "age regression" harmful habit patterns, i.e., masturbation, faulty attitudes toward sex and pregnancy, personality disorders consisting of extreme hostility toward her parents, younger brother, husband, and daughter were discovered. Posthypnotic suggestions were given and followed and the patient was reorientated to her present chronologic age.

When she had successfully passed this phase, she was then prepared for the analytic, or second part of the hypnoanalysis. This consisted of free association which indicated her fear of disapproval and punishment by her father, her extremely sensitive nature, inadequate sexual knowledge, and lack of gratification. Free association became exceedingly easy once the resistances were disintegrated through hypnosis. Hence, orthodox psychoanalytic methods benefit from this simple effective spur. Her dreams were interpreted and handled as in an analysis. In addition, the dreams described in the hypnotic state were full of pertinent details, and their significance could be easily ascertained.

Now the patient was ready for the final phase. This involved the reintegration of material derived from the hypnotic sessions. It concerned the synthesizing and redistributing of the psychological processes formerly exploited by the symptom complex. During this final phase, posthypnotic suggestions were utilized to engraft new healthy attitudes toward sexual matters and the males in her family. She realized her unconscious hostility toward her father. She had feared him because he beat her and criticized her from childhood and kept her ignorant of sex until her wedding night. This inadequate preparation for marriage also heightened the expectation of damage to her genitals. Her headaches began immediately after the brother entered the family constellation. He became her responsibility, and her father whipped her when anything happened to him. In contradistinction to her mental faculties and lack of attractiveness, the brother was brilliant and handsome. This produced additional early unconscious resentment toward males. The transition toward males was only partially accomplished by her marriage. The husband symbolized her father, causing further persistent unconscious anxieties regarding heterosexual activity. As a result of this "insight" the symptomatic meaning of her basic emotional problems became clearer. She realized that the headaches were due to her repressed hostility. They always occurred after intense emotional upsets. The lower abdominal pains, dysmenorrhea, and other psychosomatic symptoms were the "organ language" she used to verbalize for her neurosis: the frigidity. A complete change in this patient's personality occurred. All thoughts of suicide disappeared.

CASE 2. Mrs. G. N., aged 22 years. History of lumbosacral backache and throbbing pain in left leg and knee. Past medical history was essentially negative. Patient stated that following the birth of her baby six weeks ago, she developed a pain in the lower part of her back. She had a rapid and painless two and one-half hour labor under nembutal analgesia. By the tenth day the backache was so severe she could not leave the hospital. Orthopedic consultation and x-rays of the lumbosacral spine were negative. The following therapy was instituted: opiates, physiotherapy, deep x-ray therapy, paravertebral procaine injections, direct infiltration of the sciatic nerve and traction. After six weeks of this treatment the patient still complained bitterly of pain in the back and left leg. Neurological consultation was negative. A tentative diagnosis of an intervertebral disc was made and a spinogram advised. Physical examination revealed a marked scoliosis due to considerable muscle spasm on the left side.

The constant unrelieved pain indicated a psychogenic origin. The patient was very intelligent and hypnoanalysis was advised. The first few sessions were devoted to conditioning her in hypnosis. Under somnambulism the patient was able to touch the floor without pain and the scoliosis and muscle spasm disappeared. Free association revealed that she expected to have the "pains of labor" which were absent during her confinement. Therefore, she felt she had missed something. After this session she felt much better. She was told not to consider herself cured until the basic emotional difficulties were resolved. During the next two hypnotic sessions she stated that her backache recurred when she saw her mother-in-law, and that she did not want to have this baby. When two months pregnant her former employer, whom she admired, died. This resulted in an attack of severe nausea and vomiting. This man was the antithesis of her husband with whom sexual relations had always been unsatisfactory. "Even though my husband, whom I love, is very considerate, I wish he would be more firm and masculine. My old boss was handsome, ambitious, meticulous, and just perfect in every way. I wanted to name my baby after him and my husband objected and became very angry. Perhaps if I probe a little deeper I will find the reason for my backache." This was an acknowledgment that an underlying unconscious conflict existed. She refused to believe that the baby belonged to her; also, the baby, being an intruder, would break up her marital relationship. She had not seen the baby since she left the hospital. She realized the backache would not clear up permanently until she consciously solved her conflict. She was left in a deep hypnotic state for three hours and told to review all the events leading up to the present. Amnesia for this session was induced. She was to reveal the results at the next session.

It was suggested that she leave her mother-in-law's home and return to her own home. Immediately on seeing her baby she began to vomit. The nausea and vomiting were so severe that she was hospitalized. Physical examination and a flat plate of the abdomen were negative. This vomiting was a rejection or "spitting at the unwanted baby." After three days of symptomatic therapy she left the hospital still complaining of her backache and walking with considerable difficulty. Scoliosis and muscle spasm were still present.

Deep hypnosis was instituted at the next session. She realized she had not been in love with her husband, but was actually in love with her dead employer. She wished that the latter could have been the father of the baby, and this accounted for her refusal to accept the child. She had never had an orgasm with her husband. She never complained of the frigidity because she did not know to whom to turn. She now realized that the backache was an alibi for her present unhappy marital status. Also it was foolish to be in love with a dead man. She decided a more healthy attitude toward her husband was possible.

The next few visits were devoted to integrating and synthesizing repressed material into her consciousness. This resulted in the acceptance of the baby, and for the first time in her life she experienced pleasure during intercourse. She felt that "a load had been taken off her back." Her backache completely disappeared and the symptom complex of frigidity had resolved itself.

DISCUSSION OF THE HYPNOANALYTICAL METHOD

Under hypnoanalysis the patient's thoughts (free association) are spontaneous and unfold with ease. The freedom of behavior in a permissive atmosphere illustrates one of the most important aspects of hypnoanalysis. A wide latitude of expression is produced. The patient is not subservient, unconscious, or helpless. During age regression the patient's actions show the vividness with which she relives traumatic experiences. This "abreactive method" is a reliving of original experiences which takes place in her consciousness. The patient's recognition and reliving of old behavior patterns is the way she obtains "insight." She must understand the origin and the basis of her symptoms, how they are linked up with life's experiences, childhood pattern formations, and unnatural inhibitions. The symptom complex will disappear only when its symptomatic meaning has become clear to the patient.

The ego of the patient with its resistances and defenses is involved when hypnoanalysis is utilized, therefore the therapist has direct access to unconscious material. The insight gained is assimilated into the ego, and a significant change takes place. Hence, contrary to current Freudian opinion, the cure obtained through hypnoanalysis *is permanent.* No objection to the use of hypnoanalysis can be made because direct suggestion is not used.

The hypnotic technique is more rapid because the resistances are by-passed. It operates directly upon the conflict and, if solved, much of the defenses will spontaneously disappear. However, paradoxically this technique does not always require that the patient communicate or become aware of unconscious strivings. Consequently, two of our patients did not require that the unconscious be made conscious. They were able to find psychotherapeutic relief from symptoms without conscious exploration of the unconscious sources of their conflicts. Apparent recovery can take place in some patients with partial or even no insight. The patient is only interested in recovery.

What is the value of psychotherapy which does not require conscious insight? How important is the matter of making the unconscious conscious? M. H. Erickson reports two cases treated in which there is no history, no free association, no clear statements of the patient's problems, no transference, and yet a therapeutic result was achieved. Is symptomatic relief the criterion of successful psychotherapy? If the patient should be made aware of previously unknown unconscious strivings, is it necessary that she know all the steps through which her insight is achieved? More results must be evaluated before these questions are answered.

With the advent of hypnoanalysis it no longer need defend itself against the charge that hypnosis is "nothing but suggestion." The methods described present a means of accomplishing vastly more in the way of psychogynecic rehabilitation than the older methods of symptomatic relief. This study points a way to research toward a therapy which may utilize all that has been learned by the gynecologist, hypnotherapist, and psychoanalyst.

FRIGIDITY

In taking up this symptom complex we must bear in mind that we are concerned with *true* frigidity, as differentiated from pseudo-frigidity caused by ignorance and misconceptions about sexual matters, incorrect technique, or male impotence.

True frigidity may be defined as "the incapacity of women to have a vaginal orgasm." R. R. Knight states that "gynecologists and psychiatrists are aware that perhaps 75 percent of all married women derive little or no pleasure from the sexual act, and that many not only experience no pleasure, but actually suffer revulsion and pain." This fact assumes added significance from a sociological and religious aspect because of increasing extramarital promiscuity and our high divorce rate.

We feel that hypnoanalysis, a modification of hypnosis, is a rational and effective form of psychotherapy because less time and training are required. This modern and scientific method of therapy has been utilized in gynecology and obstetrics and other branches of medicine. The experimental work of numerous investigators has shown that the objections to hypnosis as a therapeutic procedure can be eradicated by utilizing hypnoanalysis following the technique described above.

E. Bergler maintains "that a typical frigid woman does not suffer from a deficiency of libido, but from a neurosis." Hence, this form of therapy is ideal for the treatment of true frigidity, because every neurosis is an illness of the unconscious. These women actually are attending a psychological masquerade, using the symptoms as a pretext for obtaining no pleasure from sexual intercourse. Nearly all of our cases presented themselves with complaints of dysmenorrhea, pelvic pain, backache, migraine headaches, and a host of other symptoms as an alibi for their lack of sexual gratification. Some of our patients had not one, but two abdominal operations without relief of the original complaint.

PSYCHOGENIC CAUSES FOR FRIGIDITY

J. P. Greenhill states "that the psychosexual factors in feminine development actually involve two organs, that the clitoris plays the dominant role in childhood." This is the most easily discovered part of the female genitalia and the one which yields the most pleasure when stimulated. Therefore, all the attention is focused upon the clitoris. This leads to suppression of the awareness of the vagina. The lack of normal pleasurable vaginal sensitivity to stimulation may be due to the denial of the vagina and the effect of pleasure seeking on the clitoris. Greenhill further states, "the other organ is the vagina, which is psychologically unimportant until puberty. In the child, the clitoris gives sexual satisfaction, while in the normal adult woman the vagina is the principal sexual organ. In frigid women, however, the transference of sexual satisfaction and excitement from the clitoris to the vagina does not take place. Hence, such women possess an infantile erotic zone, and not the adult one."

Knight states that the dynamics of this neurosis has its core in the little girl's reaction to the discovery that she is lacking in an external sexual organ possessed by the little boy, so she believes that she, too, must have once had a penis of which she was punitively deprived by the parents, or that she will somehow be given one or will grow one later. Fears, envies, and resentments proceed from the shock of this discovery, and initiate the development of conflicting hate and love toward parents, siblings, and other significant persons. Distorted sexual theories and neurotic attitudes, symptoms and personality traits derive from this source.

All investigators agree that these reactions of envy of men and fear of damage to the genitals play at least some part in the psychology of every girl, and that in many cases they are the dominating factors in personality development. Since most of the fears of mutilation, menstrual suffering, and hostile envious feelings toward men are unconscious and not to be elicited by ordinary interrogation or observations of outward behavior, we have chosen this ordinary refractory condition for treatment by hypnoanalysis.

CLASSIFICATION OF FRIGIDITY

For purposes of simplicity we may divide frigidity into two subdivisions.

A. True frigidity, founded on purely psychic mechanisms.

B. True frigidity, founded on psychophysical mechanism.

This classification excludes aplasias, hypoplasias, acquired organic lesions of the genitals, the consequences of destructive operations or accidents, incorrect technique, ignorance of sexual theories, and male impotence.

Excluded are the so-called "facultative" cases where the frigidity disappears and a normal orgasm is possible with certain men.

True frigidity on a purely psychic basis may be due to fear of punishment for violating sexual prohibitions. Again, frigidity may be due to conflicting loves, e.g., love of her father as opposed to love of her husband, love of herself as contrasted to love of her husband, and love of other women as opposed to love of men as represented by her husband. Unconscious resentments and hates with reference to a wish for revenge on men, based on the "castration" complex, or a wish to avenge the mother for all the suffering she went through at the hands of the father may also lead to frigidity.

Included are many types in whom frigidity may be easily recognized and others in whom it is more overt—who use it as an escape, a flight from their own inadequacies. In this grouping we see the homosexuals, aggressive old maids, agitative female "champions" in constant competition with males, narcissists, and violent espousers of virginity. All of these types are presumptively frigid, and their frigidity includes no physical sex factor.

In our second classification we find a "contact factor" added to our psychic disturbance. Here we see the "gold digger," who is financially exploiting many sexual partners and husbands. The prostitute and the nymphomaniac, the latter in a fruitless search for satisfaction which is never achieved, belong to this group. The members of this class may make a partial adjustment and become involved in marriage. This solves the problem only outwardly. A closer inspection will demonstrate the same pattern of flight and combat interwoven with the marriage thread. The marital union may be characterized by refusal to assume any serious obligation of wifehood or motherhood. There is an excessive compensatory interest in card playing, club and sport pursuits, and a proportionate neglect of the husband. This type will take great interest in traveling alone, purchasing expensive clothes, perhaps even the aggressive pursuit of a career. Pregnancy is avoided as a nuisance, or even a calamity.

Swinging the pendulum the other way but still within the arc of our second group, we observe those women who carry out their wifely duties with overwhelming vigor—also as an escape, and also to the exclusion of the husband. They have complete absorption in the household to the point of obsessional cleanliness and orderliness. There may be a flurry of glorified motherhood, resulting in numerous children conceived with indifference and lack of pleasure, on whom there is bestowed a surprising excess of attention and solicitude; the husband, as always, being relegated to the background. They must assume a lifetime of martyrdom, resignation, and suffering; an adoption of extreme prudishness is also not common, so that nothing but frigidity can result.

In this second grouping the physical factor is definite and demonstrable. There is no relationship between the type and degrees of frigidity and the sensitivity of the vagina.

Vaginal sensitivity may vary from complete anesthesia to exquisite receptivity. The personal attitude may range from complete revulsion, disgust, and the desire to get it over with in a hurry, to a strong sense of excitement, mounting repeatedly, but with no organismic climax and, hence, the hope for contact of long duration. The vaginal secretion may be absent, scanty, or voluminous. There may or may not be a clitoric orgasm, but never a true vaginal orgasm.

All of these possibilities, or a combination of any of them, occur in frigid women. They can occur in women with vaginismus and dyspareunia.

HYPNOANALYSIS IN FRIGIDITY

It is our contention that for the common gynecologic disorder of frigidity, hypnoanalysis is a rapid and rational form of therapy. First, because it is an illness of the unconscious (a neurosis) and not amenable to routine therapy. Second, it is masked by other symptom-equivalents, elicited only after extensive diagnostic procedures. If we are fully aware of the psychosomatic implications, if we discern the intricate psychic ramifications, how can we in all sincerity continue to treat these conditions with surgery and endocrine substitutional therapy alone? How can we approve the tediousness of classical psychoanalysis in a problem which cries out for relatively rapid relief?

Of all psychogynecic problems, none has demonstrated the efficacy and rapidity of hypnoanalysis more forcefully than the common complaint of frigidity.

RESULTS

Nine out of twelve cases of true frigidity, after a wide variety of symptomatic treatment, were permanently relieved utilizing this method. There were three failures in our limited series of cases. One patient was found to be a latent homosexual. It was decided not to attempt inversion in this case. Two other patients were not relieved following fifteen and twenty-five hours of therapy, respectively.

Two patients were permanently relieved spontaneously without any manifest reasons being revealed to the therapist. This may be due to the fact that the unconscious was made conscious of the extrapsychic conflict.

The shortest amount of time necessary to cure this symptom complex was eight hours, while the longest was sixty hours. This promising method offers a fertile field for investigators and should be evaluated by others for the ultimate welfare of psychogynecic patients of the future.

CONCLUSIONS

1. The specialties of gynecology and psychiatry overlap. Latent psychological factors (the psyche) are as responsible as the reproductive organs for many functional gynecologic conditions.

2. The vast majority of patients, especially in functional gynecologic disorders, are likely to present some psychological cause for their physiologically expressed disturbances.

3. True frigidity is a common problem in gynecology.

4. It is an illness of the unconscious; a neurosis.

5. Other gynecologic "symptom-equivalents" mask this "organ neurosis.'

6. Because of the universality of this symptom, and to obviate the division of authority, every gynecologist must be his own psychiatrist.

7. Comprehension of the psychodynamics of this symptom complex (true frigidity) must be understood.

8. Hypnoanalysis is a rational procedure in psychogynecic therapy because the recovered material is replete with significant details, new personality patterns can be engrafted, symptom-removal by direct suggestion is not utilized, and the cures, even when spontaneous, are complete and permanent.

9. Hypnoanalysis and its associative phenomena of age regression, recall of memory, free association, and posthypnotic suggestion are tremendous time-savers.

10. Hypnoanalysis varies only in degree from psychoanalysis, since it utilizes many of the concepts of the Freudian theory, i.e., interpretation of the transference, free association, piecemeal disintegration of the patient's resistances, reintegration into consciousness (assimilation by the ego) of the repressed material, and the redistribution of the psychological energies formerly exploited by the symptom complex of frigidity. Thus the patient gains insight into factors responsible for the symptom complex.

HYPNOTIC TREATMENT OF A CASE OF ACUTE HYSTERICAL DEPRESSION

BY

MILTON H. ERICKSON, M.D.

AND

LAWRENCE S. KUBIE, M.D.

An unusually capable twenty-three-year-old woman had been employed in a mental hospital for several months. Towards the end of this period she developed a progressively deepening depression. Later it became known that she had continued to discharge her duties fairly well for some weeks after a certain upsetting event; but that as time passed she had become increasingly disinterested and ineffectual in her work, slowly discontinuing all social relationships, and spending more and more time secluded in her room. At this point in her illness she ate only in response to her roommate's pleading, sobbed much of the time, occasionally expressed a wish to die, and became blocked and inhibited in speech whenever any effort was made to question her about her difficulties. During the latter part of this phase, the patient's symptoms became so acute that her relatives and friends sought psychiatric help.

The patient was seen by several psychiatrists, some of whom diagnosed her condition as the depressive phase of a manic depressive psychosis. A psychoanalyst and one of the authors, Dr. Erickson, believed it to be an acute reactive depression. Later evidence, which became available only as the story developed, indicated that it was a typical "hysterical depression," that is, a depressive reaction growing out of a definite hysterical episode.

Several consultants were in favor of commitment. To this, however, the family of the patient would not consent, insisting that some form of active psychotherapy be at least attempted. Accordingly, sympathetic and persuasive encouragement was tried. The patient responded to this sufficiently to appear slightly less depressed, and to return to her work in a feeble and rather ineffectual fashion; but she remained unable to discuss her problem.

This slight amelioration of her symptoms was sufficiently encouraging to warrant further efforts, yet was far from sufficient to free her from the danger of a relapse into deeper suicidal depression. Furthermore, the threat of commitment still hung over her head; therefore, with many misgivings the suggestion was made that she attempt psychoanalytic treatment. She showed some interest in this idea, and despite the fact that it is unusual to attempt analysis in the midst of a retarded depression, for a period of about a month she was encouraged to make daily visits to an analytically trained psychiatrist.

During this month, except for the fact that the analytic hour seemed to help the patient to make a better adjustment during the rest of the day, she made little progress, produced no free associations, related only a few fragmentary parts of her story, and usually spent the hour in depressed silence with occasional futile efforts to say something, or in sobbing as she declared that she did not know what awful thing was wrong with her or what awful thing had happened to her. Towards the end of the month she began to show signs of relapsing into an acute depression of psychotic intensity so that commitment seemed imperative.

In spite of these discouraging experiences, the family again asked that before resorting to commitment some other therapeutic measure be attempted. The suggestion that hypnotic therapy might be of value was accepted by her relatives, and plans were made for this *without the patient's knowledge*. At this point the patient's problem was referred to Dr. Erickson with the following story which had been pieced together by the various psychiatrists from the accounts of the patient's roommate, of her relatives, of a man in the case, and, in small part, of the patient herself.

CLINICAL HISTORY

The patient was the only daughter in a stern, rigid, and moralistic family. Her mother, of whom she always stood in awe, had died when the patient was thirteen years old. This had had the effect of limiting somewhat her social life, but she had an unusually close friendship with a neighbor's daughter of her own age. This friendship had continued uneventfully from childhood until the patient was twenty years old, three years before the date of the patient's illness.

At that time the two girls had made the acquaintance of an attractive young man with whom both had fallen in love. Impartial towards them at first, the young man gradually showed his preference for the other girl, and presently married her. The patient responded to this with definite disappointment and regret but quickly made an adjustment which seemed at the time to be unusually "normal," but which in view of later developments must be viewed with some suspicion. She continued her friendship with the couple, developed transitory interests in other men, and seemed to have forgotten all feelings of love for her friend's husband.

A year after the marriage, the young wife died of pneumonia. At the loss of her friend the patient showed a wholly natural grief and sorrow. Almost immediately thereafter, the young widower moved to another section of the country, and for a time dropped out of the patient's life completely. Approximately a year later he returned and by chance met the patient. Thereupon their former friendship was resumed and they began to see each other with increasing frequency.

Soon the patient confided to her roommate that she was "thinking seriously" about this man, and admitted that she was very much in love with him. Her behavior on returning from her outings with him was described by the roommate and by others as "thrilled to the skies," "happy and joyous," and "so much in love she walks on air."

One evening, after some months, she returned early and alone.

She was sobbing and her dress was stained with vomitus. To her roommate's anxious inquiries, the patient answered only with fragmentary words about being sick, nauseated, filthy, nasty and degraded. She said that love was hateful, disgusting, filthy and terrible, and she declared that she was not fit to live, that she did not want to live, and that there was nothing worth while or decent in life.

When asked if the man had done anything to her, she began to retch, renewed her sobs, begged to be left alone, and refused to permit medical aid to be summoned. Finally she yielded to persuasion and went to bed.

The next morning she seemed fairly well, although rather unhappy. She ate her breakfast, but when a friend who knew nothing of these events casually asked about the previous evening's engagement, the patient became violently nauseated, lost her breakfast, and rushed precipitously to her room. There she remained in bed the rest of the day, sobbing, uncommunicative, uncooperative with a physician who saw her, essentially repeating the behavior of the previous evening.

During that day the man tried to call on her. This precipitated another spell of vomiting; she refused to see him. She explained to her roommate that the man was "all right," but that she was nasty, filthy, disgusting and sickening, and that she would rather kill herself than ever see that man again. No additional information could be obtained from her. Thereafter, a telephone call or a letter from the man, or even the mention of his name, and finally even a casual remark by her associates about their own social contacts with men, would precipitate nausea, vomiting and acute depression.

To a psychiatrist, the man stated that on that evening they had gone for a drive and had stopped to view a sunset. Their conversation had become serious and he had told her of his love for her and of his desire to marry her. This confession he had long wanted to make, but had refrained even from hinting at it because of the recency of his wife's death and his knowledge of the depth and intimacy of the friendship that had existed between the two girls. As he had completed his confession, he had realized from the expression on her face that she reciprocated his feelings, and he had leaned over to kiss her. Immediately she had attempted to fend him off, had vomited over him in an almost projectile fashion, and had become "just plain hysterical." She had sobbed, cried, shuddered, and uttered the words "nasty," "filthy," and "degrading." By these words the man had thought she referred to her vomiting. She refused to let him take her home, seemed unable to talk to him except to tell him that she must never see him again and to declare that there was nothing decent in life. Then she had rushed frantically away.

Subsequently, all efforts on the part of friends or physicians to talk to the patient about these events had served only to accentuate the symptoms and to evoke fresh manifestations.

PREPARATION FOR AN INDIRECT HYPNOTIC INVESTIGATION

Many hints from this story induced the investigator not to attempt to hypnotize the patient simply and directly. In the first place, there was the fact that she had rejected every overt sexual word or deed with violent vomiting, and with a paralyzing depression which practically carried her out of contact with those who had attempted to help her. She rejected the man so completely that she could not hear or mention his name without vomiting; and this reaction to men had become so diffused that she could not accept the ministrations of male physicians, but reacted as though they meant to her the same kind of threat her suitor had represented. She had been able to accept him only in a spiritualized and distant courtship, or when she was protected by the presence of her friends. It was evident that she would far too greatly fear direct hypnosis to submit to it.

She was moreover too deeply entrenched in the refuge of illness to fight energetically for health. She had no resources with which to struggle against her anxiety and depression, but at any signal collapsed deeper into illness. This gave warning that in the preliminary phases of treatment one would have to work completely without her cooperation, either conscious or unconscious, without raising the least flurry of anxiety, without making a single frightening or disturbing allusion to her trouble, if possible without her even knowing that she was being inducted into treatment; and most important of all, without her feeling that the therapist (the hypnotist) was directing his conduct towards her at all. Whatever was going on in her presence must seem to her to relate to someone else. Only in this way could the treatment be undertaken with any hope of success. It should be recalled that even the passive, quiet, wordless, almost unseen presence of an analyst had been too great an aggression for the patient to accept, an intolerable erotic challenge, with the result that after a month she had sunk deeper into depression.

Accordingly, arrangements were made to have the patient's roommate confide to the patient that for some time she had been receiving hypnotic psychotherapy. Two days later the psychoanalyst approached the patient and asked her, as a favor to him in return for his efforts on her behalf, to act as a chaperone for her roommate in her regular hypnotic session with Dr. Erickson. This request he justified by the explanation that she was the only suitable chaperone who knew about her roommate's treatment, and that the nurse who usually chaperoned the treatment was unavoidably absent. The patient consented in a disinterested and listless fashion, whereupon he casually suggested that she be attentive to the hypnotic work since she herself might sometime want to try it.

By asking the patient to do this as a favor for him, the analyst put her in an active, giving role. By suggesting to her that she listen carefully because she herself might want similar help sometime, he eliminated any immediate threat, at the same time suggesting that in some undefined future she might find it useful to turn to the hypnotist for therapy.[1]

THE FIRST HYPNOTIC SESSION

Upon entering the office, the two girls were seated in adjacent chairs and a prolonged, tedious, and laborious series of suggestions were given to the roommate, who soon developed an excellent trance, thereby setting an effective example for the intended patient. During the course of this trance, suggestions were given to the roommate in such a way that by imperceptible degrees they were accepted by the patient as applying to her. The two girls were seated not far apart in identical chairs, and in such a manner that they adopted more or less similar postures as they faced the hypnotist; also they were so placed that inconspicuously the hypnotist could observe either or both of them continuously. In this way it was possible to give a suggestion to the roommate that she inhale or exhale more deeply, so timing the suggestion as to coincide with the patient's respiratory movements. By repeating this carefully many times, it was possible finally to see that any suggestion given to the roommate with regard to her respiration was automatically performed by the patient as well. Similarly, the patient having been observed placing her hand on her thigh, the suggestion was given to the roommate that she place her hand upon her thigh and that she should feel it resting there. Such maneuvers gradually and cumulatively brought the patient into a close identification with her roommate, so that gradually anything said to the roommate applied to the patient as well.

Interspersed with this were other maneuvers. For instance, the hypnotist would turn to the patient and say casually, "I hope you are not getting too tired waiting." In subsequent suggestions to the roommate that she was becoming tired, the patient herself would thereupon feel increasing fatigue without any realization that this was because of a suggestion which had been given to her. Gradually, it then became possible for the hypnotist to make suggestions to the roommate, while looking directly at the patient, thus creating in the patient an impulse to respond, just as anyone feels when someone looks at one, while addressing a question or a comment to another person.

At the expiration of an hour and a half, the patient fell into a deep trance.

Several things were done to insure her cooperation in this trance and its continuance, and to make sure that there would be opportunities to use hypnotic treatment in the future. In the first place, the patient was told gently that she was in a hypnotic trance. She was reassured that the hypnotist would do nothing that she was unwilling to have him do, and that therefore there was no need for a chaperone. She was told that she could disrupt the trance if the hypnotist should offend her. Then she was told to continue to sleep deeply for an indefinite time, listening to and obeying only every legitimate command given her by the hypnotist. Thus she was given the reassuring but illusory feeling that she had a free choice. Care was taken to make sure that she had a friendly feeling towards the hypnotist, and for future purposes a promise was secured from her to develop a deep trance at any future time for any legitimate purpose. These preliminaries were time-consuming but they were vitally necessary for safeguarding and facilitating the work to be done.

It was obvious that the patient's problems centered around emotions so violent that any therapeutic exploration would have to be carried out in some wholly "safe" fashion without provoking the least trace of guilt or fear. Such "safe exploration" meant dealing with everything in such a way that the patient could escape all painful implications. The first maneuver was to lead the patient back to a childhood devoid of childhood pain.

Accordingly, emphatic instructions were given to the patient "to forget absolutely and completely many things," carefully omitting to specify just what was to be forgotten. Thus the patient and the hypnotist entered into a tacit agreement that some things were best forgotten—that is, best repressed. Permission also was thereby given to the patient to repress them without naming them. The exploratory process which lay ahead would be facilitated by this permission to repress the more painful things, since automatically it would be applied to those which were most troublesome.[2]

Next, the patient was systematically subjected to a gradual disorientation for time and place, and then gradually was reoriented to a vaguely defined period in childhood lying somewhere between the ages of ten and thirteen. The technique used is described in some detail in studies on the hypnotic induction of color blindness and of hypnotic deafness.[3, 4] The hypnotist suggests first, a state of general confusion as to the exact day, carrying this over step by step to include the week, the month, and the year. Then this is elaborated towards an intensification of a desire to recall certain unspecified things which had occurred in previous years which also are left indeterminate. The process is a slow one and involves jumping from one confusing idea to another until out of the state of general confusion the patient develops an intense need for some definite and reassuring feeling of certainty about something, whereupon he becomes only too glad to accept definite reassurance and definite   . commands.

In reorienting the patient towards the age period between ten and thirteen, the hypnotist was careful to be extremely dogmatic in tone of voice, but equally vague and indefinite as to his precise meaning. The suggestions were given to the patient as though talking to someone else rather than directly to her. She was not told that she herself had to seize upon some meaningful event in those three years.

The years from ten to thirteen were chosen with the idea that they just preceded her mother's death, and that they must have included the period of onset of her menstruation and therefore have meant the critical turning point in her general emotional life and in her psychosexual development. Since nothing was known in detail about her life, the exact period of time to which she would finally become reoriented was left to the force of her own experiences.

She was at no time asked to name and identify specifically the age to which she became reoriented in the trance. By allowing her to avoid this specific detail, she was compelled to do something more important, namely, to speak in general terms of the total experience which those years had meant.[5]

Presently in her trance the patient showed by the childishness of her posture and manner, as well as by the childishness of her replies to casual remarks, that she had really regressed to a juvenile level of behavior. She was then told emphatically, "You know many things now, things you can never forget no matter how old you grow, and you are going to tell me those things now just as soon as I tell you what I'm talking about." These instructions were repeated over and over again with admonitions to obey them, to understand them fully, to be prepared to carry them out exactly as told, and she was urged to express and affirm her intention to carry through all of these suggestions. This was continued until her general behavior seemed to say, "Well, for what are we waiting? I'm ready."

She was told to relate everything that she knew about sex, especially in connection with menstruation, everything and anything that she had learned or been told about sex during the general period of this hypnotically reestablished but purposely undefined period in her childhood. It is fair to call this an "undefined period in her childhood" because three or four years is indeed a long time to a child, and from among the many and diverse experiences of those years she was at liberty to select those things which were of outstanding importance. Had she been confined to a more restricted span of time she could have chosen inconspicuous items. Leaving her to select from within a certain broad but critical period in her life forced her to choose the important and painful items.

Up to this point the hypnotic procedure had been systematically planned, with the expectation that any further procedure would depend upon the results of these preliminary maneuvers.

To these instructions the patient reacted with some fright. Then in a tense and childlike fashion she proceeded obediently to talk in brief disconnected sentences, phrases and words. Her remarks related to sexual activity, although in the instructions given to her emphasis had been laid not upon intercourse but upon menstruation. The following constitutes an adequate account:

"My mother told me all about that. It's nasty. Girls mustn't let boys do anything to them. Not ever. Not nice. Nice girls never do. Only bad girls. *It would make mother sick.*[6] Bad girls are disgusting. I wouldn't do it. You mustn't let them touch you. You will get nasty feelings. You mustn't let them touch you. You will get nasty feelings. You mustn't touch yourself. Nasty. Mother told me never, never, and I won't. Must be careful. Must be good. Awful things happen if you aren't careful. Then you can't do anything. It's too late. I'm going to do like mother says. She wouldn't love me if I didn't."

Many of the remarks were repeated many times in essentially identical wordings. Some were uttered only once or twice. She was allowed to continue her recitation until no new material was forthcoming, except the one additional item that this moralistic lecture had been given by the mother on several occasions.

No attempt was made to introduce any questions while she was talking, but when she had ceased she was asked, "Why does your mother tell you these many things?"

"So I'll *always* be a good girl," was the simple, earnest, childlike reply.[7]

Although it was clear, almost from the start, that the patient's passive and submissive dependence upon the mother's commands would have to be broken, it was equally evident that the image of the dead mother played a role in her life which overshadowed that

of any living person and that this idolized superego figure could
not be dislodged from its position by any direct frontal attack. For
this reason, the hypnotist's stratagem was to adopt a point of view
as nearly identical with the mother as he could. He had first to
identify himself entirely with this mother image. Only at the end
did he dare to introduce a hint of any qualifying reservations.
Therefore he began by giving the patient immediate and emphatic
assurance: "Of course you *always* will be a good girl." Then in a
manner which was in harmony with the mother's stern, rigid, moralistic, and forbidding attitudes (as judged from the patient's
manner and words), each idea attributed to the mother was carefully reviewed in the same terms, and each was earnestly approved.
In addition, the patient was admonished urgently to be glad that
her mother had already told her so many of those important things
that every mother really should tell her little girl. Finally, she was
instructed to "remember telling me about all of these things, because
I'm going to have you tell me about them again some other time."

The patient was gradually and systematically reoriented in terms
of her current age and situation in life, thereby reestablishing the
original hypnotic trance. However, the earlier instructions to "forget
many things" were still in effect, and an amnesia was induced and
maintained for all of the events of the hypnotically induced state
of regression. This was done in order to soften the transition from
those early memories to the present because of the intense conflict
which existed between the early maternal commands and her current
impulses.

She was prepared for the next step, however, by being told that
she would shortly be awakened from her trance and that then she
would be asked some questions about her childhood which she was
to answer fully. To have asked her in her ordinary waking state
about her sexual instructions would have been merely to repeat the
severe aggressions of all of her previous experiences with psychiatrists; but by telling her during her trance that questions about her
childhood would be asked, she was prepared to take a passive intellectual attitude towards the demand, and to obey it without consciously admitting its connection with her present problems.

As a further preparation for the next step, she was told that the
nature of the questions to be asked of her would not be explained

to her until she had awakened, and that until then it would suffice for her to know merely that the questions would deal with her childhood. Here again the hypnotist was governed by the basic principle of making all commands as general and nonspecific as possible, leaving it to the subject's own emotional needs to focus his remarks.

Finally, technical suggestions were given to the patient to the effect that she should allow herself to be hypnotized again, that she should go into a sound and deep trance, that if she had any resistances towards such a trance she would make the hypnotist aware of it *after* the trance had developed, whereupon she could then decide whether or not to continue in the trance. The purpose of these suggestions was merely to make certain that the patient would again allow herself to be hypnotized with full confidence that she could if she chose disrupt the trance at any time. This illusion of self-determination made it certain that the hypnotist would be able to swing the patient into a trance. Once in that condition, he was confident that he could keep her there until his therapeutic aims had been achieved.

Upon awakening, the patient showed no awareness of having been in a trance. She complained of feeling tired and remarked spontaneously that perhaps hypnosis might help her since it seemed to be helping her roommate. Purposely, no reply was made to this. Instead, she was asked abruptly, "Will you please tell me everything you can about any special instructions concerning sexual matters that your mother may have given you when you were a little girl?"

After a show of hesitation and reluctance, the patient began in a low voice and in a manner of rigid primness to repeat essentially the same story that she had told in the earlier regressive trance state, except that this time she employed a stilted, adult vocabulary and sentence structure, and made much mention of her mother. Her account was essentially as follows:

"My mother gave me very careful instruction on many occasions about the time I began to menstruate. Mother impressed upon me many times the importance of every nice girl protecting herself from undesirable associations and experiences. Mother made

me realize how nauseating, filthy and disgusting sex can be.
Mother made me realize the degraded character of anybody who
indulges in sex. I appreciate my mother's careful instruction of
me when I was just a little girl."

She made no effort to elaborate on any of these remarks, and was
obviously eager to dismiss the topic. When she had concluded her
account of her mother's teachings, they were systematically restated
to her without any comment or criticism. Instead they were given
full and earnest approval, and she was told that she should be most
grateful that her mother had taken advantage of every opportunity
to tell her little daughter those things every little child should
know and should begin to understand in childhood.

Following this an appointment was made for another interview
a week hence and she was hastily dismissed.

During the course of the following week, no new reactions were
noted in the patient by her roommate and the general trend of her
depressive behavior continued unchanged.

THE SECOND HYPNOTIC TRANCE

At the second appointment, the patient readily developed a deep
trance and at once was instructed to recall completely and in
chronological order the events of the previous session. She was asked
to review them in her mind silently, and then to recount them aloud
slowly and thoughtfully but without any elaboration.

Such silent review of a hypnotically repressed experience is a
necessary preparation. It insures completeness of the final recall.
It avoids uneven emphasis on separate elements in the recollection
and distorted emphasis which the subject subsequently would feel
the need of defending. It permits an initial recall in silence without
any feeling that in remembering facts the subject is also betraying
them to someone else. This facilitates the reassembling of painful
elements in the subject's memories. Finally, when the subject is
asked to tell aloud that which has just been thought through in
silence, it becomes a recounting of mere thoughts and memories,
rather than the more painful recounting of actual events. This also
helps to lessen the emotional barriers against communicating with
the hypnotist.

As the patient completed this task, her attention again was drawn to the fact that her mother had lectured her repeatedly. Then she was asked, "How old were you when your mother died?" to which she replied, "When I was thirteen." Immediately the comment was made with quiet emphasis. "Had your mother lived longer she would have talked to you many more times to give you advice; but since she died when you were only thirteen, she could not complete that task and so it became your task to complete it without her help."

Without giving the patient any opportunity either to accept this comment or to reject it, or indeed to react to it in any way, she quickly was switched to something else by asking her to give an account of the events which had occurred immediately after she had awakened from her first trance. As she completed the account, her attention was drawn to the repetitive character of her mother's lectures, and the same careful comment was made on the unfinished character of her mother's work.

It will be recalled that in the first day of hypnotic work the patient was brought back to an early period in her childhood and in this pseudoregression was asked to give an account of the sexual instructions her mother had given her. Then through a series of intermediate transitional states she was wakened, and in her waking state was asked to give an account of the same instructions, but with an amnesia for the fact that she had already told any of this to the hypnotist. In the second hypnotic treatment up to this point, the patient was promptly hypnotized and the posthypnotic amnesia for the first hypnotic experience was lifted so that she could recall all of the events of her first trance. Then she was asked to review the material which she had discussed immediately after awakening from the first trance, in short, her conscious memories of her mother's puritanical instructions. By reviewing in a trance both the events of her previous trance and the events that had occurred immediately on her waking from this trance, a direct link was established between the childhood ideas and affects and those of the previous week's adult experience. Thus the two could be contrasted and compared from her adult point of view.

The patient then was reoriented to the same period of early childhood. She was reminded of the account she had given before and was asked to repeat it. When she had done so, in terms essentially identical with those she had used in her original account, similar approving remarks were made, but this time so worded as to emphasize sharply the fact that these lectures had all been given to her in her childhood. When this seemed to be impressed upon her adequately, the suggestion was made quietly that as she grew older, her mother would have to give her additional advice, since things change as one grows older. This idea was repeated over and over, always in conjunction with the additional suggestion that she might well wonder what other things her mother would tell her as she grew older.

Immediately after this last suggestion, the patient was brought back from her pseudochildhood to an ordinary trance state. She was asked to repeat her account of the remarks she had made in the waking state. She was urged to take special care not to confuse the words she had used when fully awake with the words of the account she had given in the first pseudochildhood trance state, even though the ideas expressed were essentially the same, and even though she had both accounts freshly in her mind. This request constituted a permission to remember now in an ordinary trance the events of the second pseudochildhood trance, since this had been merely a repetition of the first, but the fact that there had been a second trance of this kind would not be recalled. Instead, the two trances would be blended into a single experience.

As before, the purpose of these devices was to bring gradually together the child's and the adult's points of view. Into her childhood perspective an element of expectation and of wondering had been introduced by the comment that as she grew older her mother would have had more to teach her. This now, was ready to be brought to bear upon the adult version of her mother's instructions which she had also given.

The blending of the two experiences served an additional technical purpose. In the first place, repetitions are necessary under hypnosis, just as they are in dream analysis or in the recounting of experiences by patients under analysis in general. Without repetitions one cannot be sure that all of the material is brought to expression; moreover, allowing the subject under hypnosis to recall both the original version and the various repetitions as though they were a single occasion, actually gives the subject something to hold back, namely, the fact that there were two or more experiences. This seems to satisfy the subject's need to withhold something, by giving him something unimportant to withhold in return for the important fact which is divulged. This the hypnotist can well afford to do, just as one can allow a baby to refuse to give up a rattle when he has already given up the butcher knife. The baby is satisfied and so is the parent.

As the patient concluded this task, her attention was drawn again to the period of her life in which her mother's lectures had been given, the repetitions of these lectures, their incompleteness, the unfinished task left to a little girl by her mother's death, and the necessity to speak to a child in simple and unqualified language before she is old enough for more complex adult understanding. Every effort was made to impress each of these specific points upon her, but always by the use of terms as general as possible.

Without giving the patient an opportunity to develop or elaborate these points, the suggestion was made that she might well begin the hitherto unrealized and unrecognized task of continuing for herself the course of sexual instruction which her mother had begun but had been unable to finish because of her death. She was urged that she might best begin this unfinished task by speculating earnestly and seriously upon what advice her mother would have given her during the years intervening between childhood and adolescence, and between adolescence and adult womanhood. As she accepted this suggestion, it was amplified by additional instructions to take into consideration all intellectual and emotional aspects, all such things as physical, psychological and emotional changes, development and growth, and most important to give full consideration to the ultimate reasonable goals of an adult woman, and to do so completely, fully, freely and without fear, and to elaborate each idea in full accord with the facts appropriate to herself.

Immediately after this instruction was given, the patient was told that upon awakening she should repeat all of the various accounts she had given in this hypnotic session, preferably in their chronological order, or else, if she chose, in any other comprehensive form which she preferred. Thereupon she was awakened.

The patient's waking account was decidedly brief. She slowly combined everything which she had said into a single, concise story. Significantly, she spoke in the past tense: "My mother attempted to give me an understanding of sex. She tried to give it to me in a way that a child such as I was could understand. She impressed upon me the seriousness of sex; also, the importance of having nothing to do with it. She made it very clear to me as a child."

This account was given with long pauses between each sentence, as though thinking profoundly. She interrupted herself several times to comment on her mother's death, and on the incompleteness of her instruction, and to remark that had her mother lived more things would have been said. Repeatedly she said, as if to herself, "I wonder how mother would have told me the things I should know now."

The examiner seized upon this last remark as a point for terminating the session and the patient was dismissed hastily. No attempt was made to guide her thoughts beyond the urgent instruction to speculate freely upon the things her mother would have told her and which she now needed to know. She was told to return in one week.

During this week the patient showed marked improvement. Her roommate reported "some crying, but of a different kind," and none of the previous depressed behavior. The patient seemed rather to be profoundly self-absorbed, absent-minded and puzzled; and much of the time she wore a thoughtful and sometimes bewildered expression. No attempt was made to establish any contact with the patient during the week.

THIRD HYPNOTIC SESSION

Promptly upon her arrival for the third session, the patient was hypnotized and instructed to review rapidly and silently within her own mind all of the events of the two previous sessions, to recall the instructions and suggestions which had been given to her and the responses which she had made, to include in her review any new attitudes which she might have developed and to give full and free rein to her thinking, and finally to summarize aloud her ideas and conclusions as she proceeded with this task.

Slowly and thoughtfully, but with an appearance of ease and comfort, the patient proceeded to review these events freely, briefly, and with no assistance. Her final statement summarized her performance most adequately:

"As you might say that mother tried to tell me the things I needed to know, that she would have told me how to take care of myself happily and how to look forward confidently to the time when I could do those things appropriate to my age, have a husband and a home and be a woman who has grown up."

The patient was asked to repeat this review in greater detail, in order to be sure that towards both her childhood and adult years she had achieved suitable adult attitudes. As these instructions were repeated slowly and emphatically, the patient became profoundly absorbed in thought, and, after a short while, turned with an alert, attentive expression, as if awaiting the next step.

Instruction was given that when she awoke she was to have a complete amnesia for all three sessions, including even the fact that she had been hypnotized, with the exception that she would be able to recall her first stilted, prim, waking account. This amnesia was to include any new and satisfying understanding she had come to possess. She was told further that upon awakening she would be given a systematic review of her sex instruction as the hypnotist had learned about these matters from her, but that because of the all-inclusive amnesia this review would seem to her to be a hypothetical construction of probabilities built by the hypnotist upon that first waking account. As this occurred, she was to listen with intense interest and evergrowing understanding. She would find truths and meanings and applications understandable only to her in whatever was said and, as those continued and developed, she would acquire a capacity to interpret, to apply and to recognize them as actually belonging to her, and to do so far beyond any capacity that the hypnotist might have to understand.

At first glance, it would seem strange to suggest repression of insight as one of the culminating steps in a therapeutic procedure. In the first place, it implies that much of the affective insight may either remain or again become unconscious without lessening its therapeutic value. Secondly, it protects the subject from the dis-

turbing feeling that anyone else knows the things about her which
she now knows, but which she wishes to keep to herself; hence the
importance of the suggestion that she would understand far more
than the hypnotist. Thirdly, by looking upon the material as a
purely hypothetical construction of probabilities by the hypnotist,
the patient was provided with an opportunity to recover insight
gradually in a slowly progressive fashion as she tested this hypothetical structure. Had the same material been presented to her
as definite and unquestionable facts, she might again have developed
sudden repressions with a spontaneous loss of all insight. If that
occurred, the investigation would have had to be undertaken afresh.
On the other hand, where a certain measure of repression is ordered
by the hypnotist, it remains under his control, because what the
hypnotist suppresses he can recover at will. Thus her degree of
insight remained under full and complete control by the hypnotist,
so that he could at any time give the patient full insight, or prepare
her for it again. Finally, by depriving the patient temporarily of
her new and gratifying insight, a certain unconscious eagerness and
need for further knowledge was developed which assisted in the
ultimate recovery of full insight.

When these instructions had been repeated sufficiently to effect
a full understanding, the patient was awakened with an amnesia
for all events except the stilted prim account which she had given
at the end of the first therapeutic session. Reminding her of that
account the hypnotist offered to speculate upon the probable nature
and development of the sex instructions which she had been given.
He proceeded to review all the material she had furnished in general
terms that permitted her to apply them freely to her own experiences.

Thus the patient was given a general review of the development
of all of the primary and secondary sexual characteristics: the
phenomenon of menstruation, the appearance of pubic and axillary
hair, the development of her breasts, the probable interest in the
growth of her nipples, the first wearing of a brassiere, the possibilities that boys had noticed her developing figure and that some of
them may have slapped her freshly, and the like. Each was named
in rapid succession without placing emphasis on any individual
item. This was followed by a discussion of modesty, of the first feelings of sexual awareness, of autoerotic feelings, of the ideas of love

in puberty and adolescence, of the possible ideas of where babies came from. Thus without any specific data, a wide variety of ideas and typical experiences were covered by name. After this, general statements were made as to the speculations that might have passed through her mind at one time or another. This again was done slowly and always in vague general terms, so that she could make a comprehensive and extensive personal application of these remarks.

Shortly after this procedure was begun the patient responded by a show of interest and with every outward manifestation of insight and of understanding. At the conclusion the patient declared simply, "You know, I can understand what has been wrong with me, but I'm in a hurry now and I will tell you tomorrow."

This was the patient's first acknowledgment that she had a problem and instead of permitting her to rush away she was promptly rehypnotized, and was emphatically instructed to recover any and all memories of her trance experiences that would be of use. By stressing in this way the fact that certain of those memories would be valuable and useful to her, the patient was led to view all of them as possibly useful, thus withdrawing her attention from any conflicting feelings about those memories. This assists in their free and full recovery by the patient. She was told that she should feel free to ask for advice, suggestions and any instruction that she wished, and to do so freely and comfortably. As soon as this instruction had been firmly impressed, the patient was awakened.

Immediately, but with less urgency, she said that she wanted to leave but added that she would first like to ask a few questions. When told that she might do so, the patient asked the hypnotist to state his personal opinion about "kissing, petting, and necking." Very cautiously and using her own words, approbation was given of all three, with the reservation that each should be done in a manner which conformed with one's own ideals and that only such amorous behavior could be indulged in as would conform to the essential ideals of the individual personality. The patient received this statement thoughtfully, and then asked for a personal opinion as to whether it was right to feel sexual desires. The cautious reply was given that sexual desire was a normal and essential feeling for every living creature and that its absence from appropriate situations was wrong. To this was added the statement that she would undoubtedly agree that her own mother, were she living, would have said the same thing. After thinking this over, the patient left hastily.

THERAPEUTIC OUTCOME

The next day the patient returned to declare that she had spent the previous evening in the company of her suitor. With many blushes she added, "Kissing is great sport." Thereupon she made another hurried departure.

A few days later she was seen by appointment and held out her left hand to display an engagement ring. She explained that as a result of her talk with the hypnotist during the last therapeutic session, she had gained an entirely new understanding of many things, and that this new understanding had made it possible for her to accept the emotion of love and to experience sexual desires and feelings, and that she was now entirely grown up and ready for the experiences of womanhood. She seemed unwilling to discuss matters further, except to ask whether she might have another interview with the hypnotist in the near future, explaining that at that time she would like to receive instruction about coitus, since she expected to be married shortly. She added with some slight embarrassment, "Doctor, that time I wanted to rush away. . . . By not letting me rush away, you saved my virginity. I wanted to go right to him and offer myself to him at once."

Sometime later she was seen in accordance with her request. A minimum of information was given her and it was found that she had no particular worries or concern about the entire matter and was straightforward and earnest about her desire to be instructed. Shortly afterwards the patient came in to report that she was to be married within a few days and that she looked forward happily to her honeymoon.

About a year later she came in to report that her married life was all she could hope for, and that she was anticipating motherhood with much pleasure. Two years later she was seen again and was found to be happy with her husband and her baby daughter.

SUMMARY AND DISCUSSION

For special reasons the treatment of this patient had to be approached with many precautions. The circumstances of her illness made a direct approach to her problem (whether by a man or a woman) dangerous because such an approach invariably caused an acute increase of her panic and of her suicidal depression. She could be treated, if at all, only by creating an elaborate pretense of leaving her problems quite alone, without even letting her realize that any therapy was being attempted, without acknowledging the development of a relationship between the patient and the physician, and without open reference to the experiences which had precipitated her illness.

For these reasons, the treatment was begun by pretending to treat someone else in her presence, and through this means, she was slowly and gradually brought into a hypnotic state in which her own problems could be approached more directly.

From this point on the treatment proceeded along lines which are the reverse of the usual psychoanalytic technique. Some points seem to be worthy of special emphasis.

Instead of depending solely upon memory to recover important experiences out of the past, the patient under hypnosis was translated back to a critical period of her childhood, so that in this state she could relive or revive the general quality of the influences playing upon her, but without recapturing the details of specific scenes and episodes. Instead of stirring them up and making them conscious, there was a deliberate effort to avoid the induction of any feelings of guilt or fear. Similarly, instead of insisting upon total conscious recall, permission was freely granted to the patient to forget painful things, not only during but also after the hypnotic treatment. Underlying this permission to forget was the confidence that even those facts which were consciously forgotten could be recovered during the hypnosis when needed for therapeutic use, and that their therapeutic efficacy would continue even during the posthypnotic repression.

The hypnotist's attack on the patient's rigid superego was interesting from various points of view. Particularly noteworthy, however, was the fact that the attack on the superego began with a complete support of all of the most repressive attitudes which the patient attributed to her dead mother. It was only by forming a bond in this way between himself and the mother that he was able later slowly to undermine the rigidity of this repressive figure and thus to penetrate the patient's tense and automatic defenses of her mother's dictates. Another significant point is the method used by the hypnotist to help the patient silently to assemble her ideas before communicating them. This seemed to assist materially in reducing the patient's fear of remembering presumably because it is not as difficult to recall embarrassing things which one can keep to one's self, as it is to bring them to mind with the knowledge that one must confess them at once; moreover, once such things have been reviewed in thought, it becomes easier to talk of the thoughts than it would have been to talk of the events themselves. This two-stage method of recalling and assembling data before communicating it might have its usefulness in analysis as well.

A point at which the work of the hypnotist coincides closely with that of the analyst is in the use of repetitions in many forms and at each age level investigated. This use of repetitions is quite similar to what is found to be necessary in analysis as well.

In understanding the course of this treatment and of the patient's recovery, there are many gaps in the material, gaps which could be filled in only by conducting a treatment of this kind in a patient who had been under a fairly prolonged analysis.

There are many questions we would like to have answered. Was the basis of the mother's overwhelming authority primarily affection or hostility and fear? Were the dead mother and the dead friend equivalent? If the hypnotist had said instead that he was the dear friend, and that as the dead friend he encouraged and approved of her lovemaking with the dead friend's husband (an equivalent of a mother telling her that she could make love to her father), would this impersonation of the friend by the hypnotist have freed the patient from guilt feelings and from her hysterical depression without the induced regression to childhood? What was the mechanism of the cure? Was the hypnotist equated to her mother, and thus enabled to remove the mother's taboos? Or was the fiancé at first a surrogate father until the hypnotist took over the father's role, thus removing it from the man, and thereby making it possible for the patient to have an erotic relation with the man without a barrier of incest taboos? What was the role of her orality and its significance in relationship to the vomiting? In general, what was the role of all of those basic facts of her early life which must have determined the patient's relationship to her parents and to people in general?

The answers to these gaps in information is challenging, both from a theoretical and from a factual point of view. The knowledge of these facts is indispensable for an understanding of the structure of the illness and the dynamics of the recovery. But the fact that recovery could take place so quickly and without hospitalization, in face of the fact that there were so many things which the hypnotist never discovered and that the patient did not know, also has its important theoretical consequences. It faces us with the question: if recovery can take place with the gain of such rudimentary insight, what then is the relationship between unconscious insight, conscious insight, and the process of recovery from a neurosis?

HYPNOTIC PSYCHOTHERAPY

MILTON H. ERICKSON, M.D.

Since the most primitive times, hypnosis has been employed almost universally in the practice of religious and medical rites to intensify belief in mysticism, magic and medicine. The impressive bewildering character of hypnotic manifestations and the profoundly inexplicable, seemingly miraculous, psychological effects upon human behavior achieved by the use of hypnosis, have served to bring about two general contradictory attitudes toward it. The first of these is the unscientific attitude of superstitious awe, fear, disbelief and actual hostility, all of which have delayed and obstructed the growth of scientific knowledge of hypnosis.

The second attitude is one of scientific acceptance of hypnosis as a legitimate and valid psychological phenomenon, of profound importance and significance in the investigation and understanding of human behavior, and of the experiential life of the individual. This attitude had its first beginnings with the work of Anton Mesmer in 1775, who tempered his scientific approach to an understanding of hypnosis by mystical theories. Nevertheless, Mesmer did succeed in demonstrating the usefulness and effectiveness of hypnosis in the treatment of certain types of patients otherwise unresponsive to medical care. Thus he laid the foundation for the therapeutic use of hypnosis and for the recognition of psychotherapy as a valid psychological medical procedure.

Since then there has been a long succession of clinically trained men who demonstrated the usefulness of hypnosis as a therapeutic medical procedure and as a means of examining, understanding and reeducating human behavior. Among these was James Braid, a Scotch physician who, in 1841, first discredited the superstitious mystical ideas about the nature of hypnosis, or "mesmerism," as it was then called. Braid recognized the phenomenon as a normal psychological manifestation, coined the terms of "hypnosis" and "hypnotism," and devised a great variety of scientific experimental studies to determine its medical and psychological values.

Following Braid, many outstanding scientists, including both clinicians and later psychologists, accepted his findings and contributed increasingly to the scientific development of hypnosis despite the hampering heritage of traditional misconceptions, fears and hostilities that have surrounded it and still do among the uninformed.

During the past twenty-five years there have been an increasing number of studies demonstrating hypnosis to be of outstanding value in investigating the nature and structure of personality, in understanding normal and abnormal behavior, in studying interpersonal and intrapersonal relationships and psychosomatic interrelationships. Also, there have been extensive developments in the utilization of hypnosis as an effective instrument for psychotherapy.

Any discussion of hypnotic psychotherapy or hypnotherapy requires an explication of general consideration derived from clinical observation. The following observations and case history indicate some of the misconceptions, oversights and difficulties of hypnotherapy; and also illustrate various technics and explanations of their use which are conducive to effective application of this therapeutic tool.

DIFFERENTIATION BETWEEN TRANCE INDUCTION AND TRANCE STATE

One of the first considerations in undertaking hypnotic psychotherapy centers around the differentiation of the patient's experience of having a trance induced from the experience of being in a trance state. As an analogy, the train trip to the city is one order of experience; being in the city is another. To continue, the process of

inducing a trance should be regarded as a method of teaching the
patient a new manner of learning something, and thereby enabling
him to discover unrealized capacities to learn, and to act in new
ways which may be applied to other and different things. The importance of trance induction as an educational procedure in
acquainting the patient with his latent abilities has been greatly
disregarded.

Both the therapist and the patient need to make this differentiation, the former in order to guide the patient's behavior more
effectively, the latter in order to learn to distinguish between his
conscious and unconscious behavior patterns. During trance induction, the patient's behavior is comprised of both conscious and unconscious patterns, while the behavior of the trance state should
be primarily of unconscious origin.

The failure of such distinction or differentiation between the induction and the trance often results in the patient's attempting to
perform the work of the trance state in the same fashion as he
learned to develop a trance. That is, without proper differentiation,
the patient will utilize both conscious and unconscious behavior in
the trance instead of relying primarily upon unconscious patterns of behavior. This leads to inadequate faulty task performance.

Although patients can, and frequently do, make this distinction
spontaneously, the responsibility, though often overlooked, rests
properly with the therapist. To insure such differentiation, the
trance induction should be emphasized as a preparation of the patient for another type of experience in which new learnings will be
utilized for other purposes and in a different way. This education of
the patient can be achieved best, as experience has shown, by teaching him how to become a good hypnotic subject, familiar with all
types of hypnotic phenomena. This should be done before any attempt is made at therapy. Such training, while it postpones the
initiation of direct therapy, actually hastens the progress of therapy
since it gives the patient wider opportunities for self-expression.
For example, the patient who can develop hypnotic hallucinations,
both visual and auditory, manifest regressive behavior, do automatic
writing, act upon posthypnotic suggestions, and dream upon command is in an advantageous position for the reception of therapy.

As for the trance state itself, this should be regarded as a special, unique, but wholly normal psychological state. It resembles sleep only superficially, and it is characterized by various physiological concomitants, and by a functioning of the personality at a level of awareness other than the ordinary or usual state of awareness. For convenience in conceptualization, this special state, or level of awareness, has been termed "unconscious" or "subconscious." The role in hypnotic psychotherapy of this special state of awareness is that of permitting and enabling the patient to react, uninfluenced by his conscious mind, to his past experiential life and to a new order of experience which is about to occur as he participates in the therapeutic procedure. This participation in therapy by the patient constitutes the primary requisite for effective results.

ROLE OF SUGGESTION IN HYPNOSIS

The next consideration concerns the general role of suggestion in hypnosis. Too often, the unwarranted and unsound assumption is made that, since a trance state is induced and maintained by suggestion, and since hypnotic manifestations can be elicited by suggestion, whatever develops from hypnosis must necessarily be completely a result of suggestion and primarily an expression of it. Contrary to such misconceptions, the hypnotized person remains the same person. His behavior only is altered by the trance state, but even so, that altered behavior derives from the life experience of the patient and not from the therapist. At the most, the therapist can influence only the manner of self-expression. The induction and maintenance of a trance serve to provide a special psychological state in which the patient can reassociate and reorganize his inner psychological complexities and utilize his own capacities in a manner in accord with his own experiential life. Hypnosis does not change the person nor does it alter his past experiential life. It serves to permit him to learn more about himself and to express himself more adequately.

Direct suggestion is based primarily, if unwittingly, upon the assumption that whatever develops in hypnosis derives from the suggestions given. It implies that the therapist has the miraculous power of effecting therapeutic changes in the patient, and disregards the fact that therapy results from an inner resynthesis of the patient's behavior achieved by the patient himself. It is true that direct suggestion can effect an alteration in the patient's behavior and result in a symptomatic cure, at least temporarily. However, such a "cure" is simply a response to the suggestion and does not entail that reassociation and reorganization of ideas, understandings and memories so essential for an actual cure. It is this experience of reassociating and reorganizing his own experiential life that eventuates in a cure, not the manifestation of responsive behavior which can, at best, satisfy only the observer.

For example, anesthesia of the hand may be suggested directly and a seemingly adequate response may be made. However, if the patient has not spontaneously interpreted the command to include a realization of the need for inner reorganization, that anesthesia will fail to meet clinical tests and will be a pseudo-anesthesia.

An effective anesthesia is better induced, for example, by initiating a train of mental activity within the patient himself by suggesting that he recall the feeling of numbness experienced after a local anesthetic, or after a leg or arm went to sleep, and then suggesting that he can now experience a similar feeling in his hand. By such an indirect suggestion the patient is enabled to go through those difficult inner processes of disorganizing, reorganizing, reassociating and projecting of inner real experience to meet the requirements of the suggestion and thus, the induced anesthesia becomes a part of his experiential life, instead of a simple, superficial response.

The same principles hold true in psychotherapy. The chronic alcoholic can be induced by direct suggestion to correct his habits temporarily, but not until he goes through the inner process of reassociating and reorganizing his experiential life can effective results occur.

In other words, hypnotic psychotherapy is a learning process for the patient, a procedure of reeducation. Effective results in hypnotic psychotherapy, or hypnotherapy, derive only from the patient's activities. The therapist merely stimulates the patient into activity, often not knowing what that activity may be, and then he guides the patient and exercises clinical judgment in determining the amount of work to be done to achieve the desired results. How to guide and to judge constitute the therapist's problem while the patient's task is that of learning through his own efforts to understand his experiential life in a new way. Such reeducation is, of course, necessarily in terms of the patient's life experiences, his understandings, memories, attitudes and ideas, and it cannot be in terms of the therapist's ideas and opinions. For example, in training a gravid patient to develop anesthesia for eventual delivery, use was made of the suggestions outlined above as suitable. The attempt failed completely even though she had previously experienced local dental anesthesia and also her legs "going to sleep." Accordingly, the suggestion was offered that she might develop a generalized anesthesia in terms of her own experiences when her body was without sensory meaning to her. This suggestion was intentionally vague since the patient, knowing the purpose of the hypnosis, was enabled by the vagueness of the suggestion to make her own selection of those items of personal experience that would best enable her to act upon the suggestion.

She responded by reviewing mentally the absence of any memories of physical stimuli during physiological sleep, and by reviewing her dreams of walking effortlessly and without sensation through closed doors and walls and floating pleasantly through the air as a disembodied spirit looking happily down upon her sleeping, unfeeling body. By means of this review, she was able to initiate a process of reorganization of her experiential life. As a result, she was able to develop a remarkably effective anesthesia, which met fully the needs of the subsequent delivery. Not until sometime later did the therapist learn by what train of thought she had initiated the neuro-psycho-physiological processes by which she achieved anesthesia.

SEPARATENESS OF CONSCIOUS AND SUBCONSCIOUS LEVELS OF AWARENESS

Another common oversight in hypnotic psychotherapy lies in the lack of appreciation of the separateness or the possible mutual exclusiveness of the conscious and the unconscious (or subconscious) levels of awareness. Yet, all of us have had the experience of having a word or a name "on the tip of the tongue" but being unable to remember it so that it remained unavailable and inaccessible in the immediate situation. Nevertheless, full knowledge actually existed within the unconscious, but unavailably so to the conscious mind.

In hypnotic psychotherapy, too often, suitable therapy may be given to the unconscious but with the failure by the therapist to appreciate the tremendous need of either enabling the patient to integrate the unconscious with the conscious, or, of making the new understandings of the unconscious fully accessible, upon need, to the conscious mind. Comparable to this failure would be an appendectomy with failure to close the incision. It is in this regard that many arm-chair critics naïvely denounce hypnotic psychotherapy as without value since "it deals only with the unconscious." Additionally, there is even more oversight of the fact, repeatedly demonstrated by clinical experience, that in some aspects of the patient's problem direct reintegration under the guidance of the therapist is desirable; in other aspects, the unconscious should merely be made available to the conscious mind, thereby permitting a spontaneous reintegration free from any immediate influence by the therapist. Properly, hypnotherapy should be oriented equally about the conscious and unconscious, since the integration of the total personality is the desired goal in psychotherapy.

However, the above does not necessarily mean that integration must constantly keep step with the progress of the therapy. One of the greatest advantages of hypnotherapy lies in the opportunity to work independently with the unconscious without being hampered by the reluctance, or sometimes actual inability, of the conscious mind to accept therapeutic gains. For example, a patient had full unconscious insight into her periodic nightmares of an incestuous character from which she suffered, but, as she spontaneously declared in the trance, "I now understand those horrible dreams, but I couldn't possibly tolerate such an understanding consciously." By this utterance, the patient demonstrated the protectiveness of the unconscious for the conscious. Utilization of this protectiveness as a motivating force enabled the patient subsequently to accept consciously her unconscious insights.

Experimental investigation has repeatedly demonstrated that good unconscious understandings allowed to become conscious before a conscious readiness exists will result in conscious resistance, rejection, repression and even the loss, through repression, of unconscious gains. By working separately with the unconscious there is then the opportunity to temper and to control the patient's rate of progress and thus to effect a reintegration in the manner acceptable to the conscious mind.

ILLUSTRATIVE CASE HISTORY

A 28-year-old married man sought therapy because he believed implicitly that he did not love his wife and that he had married her only because she resembled superficially his mother to whom he was strongly attached. In the trance state he affirmed this belief. During hypnotherapy, he learned, in the trance state, that his marital problem had arisen from an intense mother-hatred disguised as oversolicitude and that his wife's superficial resemblance to the mother rendered her an excellent target for his manifold aggressions. Any attempt to make his unconscious understandings conscious confronted him with consciously unendurable tasks of major revisions in all of his interpersonal relationships and a recognition of his mother-hatred which, to him, seemed to be both intolerable and impossible.

In psychotherapy, other than hypnotic, the handling by the patient of such a problem as this would meet with many conscious resistances, repressions, rationalizations and efforts to reject any insight. The hypnotherapeutic procedures employed to correct this problem will be given in some detail below. No attempt will be made to analyze the underlying dynamics of the patient's problem since the purpose of this paper is to explicate methods of procedure, new technics, the utilization of mental mechanisms, and the methods of guiding and controlling the patient's progress so that unconscious insight becomes consciously acceptable.

Early in the course of this patient's treatment it had been learned that he did not consciously dare to look closely at his mother, that he did not know the color of his mother's eyes, or the fact that she wore dentures, and that a description of his mother was limited to "she is so gentle and graceful in her movements, and her voice is so soft and gentle, and she has such a sweet, kind, gracious expression on her face that a miserable neurotic failure like me does not deserve all the things she has done for me."

When, during hypnotherapy, he had reached a stage at which his unconscious understandings and insights seemed to be reasonably sufficient to permit the laying of a foundation for the development of conscious understandings, he was placed in a profound somnambulistic trance. He was then induced to develop a profound amnesia for all aspects of his problem, and a complete amnesia for everything about his mother and his wife, except the realization that he must have had a mother. This amnesia included also his newly acquired unconscious understandings.

There are special reasons for the induction of such a profound amnesia or repression. One is that obedience to such a suggestion constitutes a relinquishing of control to the therapist of the patient's repression tendencies. Also, it implies to the patient that if the therapist can repress he also can restore. In undertaking hypnotherapy, it is important in the early stages to have the patient develop an amnesia for some innocuous memory, then to restore that memory along with some other unimportant but forgotten memory. Thus, an experiential background is laid for the future recovery of vital repressed material.

The other reason is that such an amnesia or induced repression clears the slate for a reassociation and reorganization of ideas, attitudes, feelings, memories and experiences. In other words, the amnesia enables the patient to be confronted with material belonging to his own experiential life but which, because of the induced repression, is not recognized by him as such. Then it becomes possible for that patient to reach a critical objective understanding of unrecognized material from his own life experience, to reorganize and reassociate it in accord with its reality significances and his own personality needs. Even though the material has been repressed from both the unconscious and the conscious, his personality needs still exist and any effort to deal with the material presented will be in relationship to his personality needs. As an analogy, the child on a calcium deficient diet knows nothing about calcium deficiency nor calcium content, but, nevertheless, shows a marked preference for calcium rich food.

After the induction of the amnesia, the next step was a seemingly casual brief discussion of the meaning of feminine names. Then it was suggested that he see, sitting in the chair on the other side of the room, a strange woman who would converse with him and about whom he would know nothing except for a feeling of firm conviction that her first name was Nelly. Previous hypnotic training at the beginning of hypnotherapy had prepared him for this type of experience.

The patient's response to that particular name, as intended, was that of an hallucination of his mother whom he could not, because of the amnesia, recognize as such. He was induced to carry on an extensive conversation with this hallucinatory figure, making many inquiries along lines pertinent to his own problem. He described her adequately and objectively. He was asked to "speculate" upon her probable life history, and the possible reasons therefor. He was asked to relate to the therapist in detail all that Nelly "said" and to discuss this material fully. Thus, careful guidance by the therapist enabled him to review objectively, critically, and with free understanding a great wealth of both pleasant and unpleasant material, disclosing his relationships to his mother and his comprehension of what he believed to be her understandings of the total situation. Thus he was placed in a situation permitting the development of a new frame of reference at variance with the repressed material of his life experience, but which would permit a reassociation, an elaboration, a reorganization and an integration of his experiential life.

In subsequent therapeutic sessions, a similar procedure was followed, separately, with two other hallucinated figures, "spoken of" by Nelly as her son Henry and his wife Madge, neither of whom the patient could recognize because of his induced amnesia.

The hypnotic session with Henry was greatly prolonged since Henry "told" the patient a great wealth of detailed information which the patient discussed with the therapist freely and easily and with excellent understanding. The patient's interview with the hallucinatory Madge was similarly conducted.

Of tremendous importance in the eventual therapeutic result was the patient's report upon the emotional behavior he "observed" in the hallucinated figures as they related their stories, and his own objective, dispassionate appraisal of "their emotions." He frequently expressed amazement to the therapist and to the hallucinated figures over "their" inability to understand "their own emotions."

To explain this procedure, it must be recognized that all of the material the patient "elicited" from the hallucinatory figures was only the projection of the repressed material of his own experience. Even though a profound repression for all aspects of his problem had been induced, that material still existed and could be projected upon others since the projection would not necessarily lead to recognition. To illustrate from everyday experience, those personality traits disliked by the self are easily repressed from conscious awareness and are readily recognized in others or projected upon others. Thus, a common mental mechanism was employed to give the patient a view of himself which could be accepted and integrated into his total understandings.

The culminating step in this procedure consisted in having him hallucinate Nelly and Henry together, Madge and Henry, Nelly and Madge, and finally all three together. Additionally, he was induced to develop each of these various hallucinations in a great number of different life settings known from his history to be traumatic, such as a shopping trip with his wife which had resulted in a bitter quarrel over a minor matter, a dinner table scene, and a quarrel between his wife and his mother.

Thus, the patient, as an observant, objective, judicious third person, through the mechanisms of repression and projection, viewed freely, but without recognition, a panorama of his own experiential life, a panorama which permitted the recognition of faults and distortions without the blinding effects of emotional bias.

In the next session, again in a profound somnambulistic trance, he was emphatically instructed to remember clearly in full detail everything he had seen, heard, thought, and speculated upon and appraised critically in relationship to Nelly, Henry and Madge. To this he agreed readily and interestedly. Next, he was told to single out various traumatic incidents and to wonder, at first vaguely, and then with increasing clarity, whether or not a comparable incident had ever occurred in his life. As he did this, he was to have the privilege of remembering any little thing necessary in his own history. Thus, he was actually given indirect instructions to break down by slow degrees the induced amnesia or repression previously established.

The patient began this task slowly, starting with the simple declaration that a cup on the table, in a dinner scene he had hallucinated, very closely resembled one he had had since childhood. He next noted that he and Henry had the same first name, and wondered briefly what Henry's last name was, then hastily observed that Madge and Henry evidently lived in the same town as he did, inasmuch as he had recognized the store in which they quarreled so foolishly. He commented on Nelly's dentures and, with some reluctance, related his fears of dentists, and of losing his teeth, and being forced to put up a "false front." As he continued his remarks, he became more and more revealing. Gradually, he tended to single out the more strongly emotional items, spacing them with intervening comments upon relatively innocuous associations. After more than an hour of this type of behavior, he began to have slips of the tongue which he would immediately detect, become tense, and then, upon reassurance by the therapist, he would continue his task. For example, in comparing Nelly's light brown eyes with Madge's dark brown eyes he made the additional comment, "My wife's eyes are like Madge's." As he concluded his statement, he showed a violent startle reaction and in a tone of intense surprise repeated questioningly, "My wife?" After a moment's hesitation, he remarked to himself "I know I'm married. I have a wife. Her name is Madge. She has brown eyes like Madge. But that is all I know. I can't remember any more— nothing—nothing!" Then, with an expression of much anxiety and fear, he turned to the therapist and asked pleadingly, "Is there something wrong with me?"

He was immediately reassured that nothing was wrong, that something very good, desirable and right was happening to him, and he was warmly praised for the excellence of the work he was doing, the courage he was showing, and the remarkable clarity of the understandings he was developing. The effect of this reassurance and praise was to make him plunge more deeply and energetically into his task.

Shortly he discovered the similarity between Nelly and his mother, and continued, with excellent understanding, by appraising Nelly as an unhappy neurotic woman deserving normal consideration and affection. This led to the sudden statement, "that applies to my mother too—Good God, Nelly is my mother only I was seeing her for the first time—her eyes are brown—like Madge's. My wife's eyes are brown—her name is Madge—Madge IS my wife."

There followed then a whole series of fragmentary remarks relating to traumatic situations, of which the following are examples:

"The fight at the store—that coat she bought—we almost broke our engagement—birthday cake—shoe string broke—Good God, what can I ever say to her?" After each utterance he seemed to be absorbed in recalling some specific, emotionally charged event in detail. After about twenty minutes of this behavior he leaned forward, cupped his chin in his hands, and lost himself in silent reflection for some minutes, terminating this by asking in a questioning manner, "Nelly, who is Nelly?" but immediately absorbed himself in reflection again. For some time longer, he sat tense and rigid, shifting his gaze rapidly here and there and apparently thinking with great feeling. About fifteen minutes later, he slowly relaxed, and, in a tired voice declared, "That was hard. Henry is me. Now I know what I've been doing, what I've been doing here, and been doing all my life. But I'm not afraid any more. I don't need to be afraid—not any more. It's an awful mess, but I know how to clean it up. And I'm going to make an appointment with the dentist. But it's all got to take a lot of thinking—an awful lot, but I'm ready to do it."

Turning to the therapist he stated, "I'm tired, awful tired."

A series of questions and answers now disclosed that the patient felt satisfied, that he felt comfortable with the rush of new understandings he had experienced, that he knew that he was in a trance, and that he was at a loss to know how to let his conscious mind learn what he now knew in his unconscious. When asked
• if he wanted some suggestions in that regard, he eagerly indicated that he did.

He was reminded of how the induced amnesia had been broken down by the slow filtering out of ideas and associations by outward projection where he could examine them without fear or prejudice and thus achieve an understanding. With each new understanding he had experienced further reorganization of his experiential life, although he could not sense it at first. This, as he could understand, was a relatively simple, easy task, and involved nothing more than himself and his thinking and feelings. To become consciously aware of his new understandings would involve himself, his thinking, his everyday activities, his own personal relationships, and the interpersonal relationships of other people. This, therefore, would be an infinitely more difficult task. Upon full understanding of this, an agreement was reached to the effect that he would continue to be neurotic in his everyday life, but, as he did so, he would slowly and gradually develop a full conscious realization of the meaningfulness of his neuroticisms, first of the very minor ones and then, as he bettered his adjustments in minor ways, to progress to the more difficult problems. Thus, bit by bit, he could integrate his unconscious learnings with his conscious behavior in a corrective fashion which would lead to good adjustment.

The above paragraph is but a brief summary of the discussion offered the patient. Although he believed he understood the explanation the first time, as experience has shown repeatedly, it is always necessary to reiterate and to elaborate from many different points of view and to cite likely incidents in which unconscious insights can break through to the conscious before the patient really understands the nature of the task before him. A possible incident was cited for him by which to learn how to let unconscious learning become conscious. On some necessary trip to the store where the quarrel had occurred he would notice some clerk looking amused at something. He would then experience a strong feeling of amusement for no known reason, wonder why, discover that his amusement was tinged with a mild feeling of embarrassment, and suddenly recall the quarrel with his wife in its true proportions, and thus lose his conscious resentments. A few other such incidents were also suggested, and, as subsequently learned, were acted upon. He was then awakened from the trance and dismissed.

The patient's first step to effect a conscious integration, in accord with his trance declaration, was to visit, with much fear, his dentist, thereby discovering, when once in the dental chair, how grossly exaggerated his fears had been. Next, he found himself humming a song while putting on his shirt, instead of examining it compulsively for wrinkles, as had been his previous habit.

Examination of all the family photographs initiated a process of identification of himself, his mother and his wife. He discovered for the first time that he resembled his father strongly and could not understand why he had previously believed so fully that he was the image of his mother. By way of the photographs, he discovered the dissimilarities between his wife and his mother, and that dentures had actually altered his mother's facial appearance.

At first, his adjustments were made singly and in minor matters, but, after a few weeks, larger and larger maladjustments were corrected. Usually, these were corrected without his conscious awareness until sometime later, a measure which had been suggested to him. For example, he had always visited his mother regularly at the hour of her favorite radio program, and he had always insisted on listening to another program which he invariably criticized unfavorably. Unexpectedly, one day, he became aware that, for several weeks, he had been making his visits at a different hour. With much amusement he realized that his mother could now listen to her favorite program, and at the same time he experienced the development of much insight into the nature of his attitudes toward his mother.

During this period of reintegration, he visited his therapist regularly, usually briefly. Sometimes his purpose was to discuss his progress consciously, sometimes to be hypnotized and given further therapy.

One of his last steps was to discover that he loved his wife and always had, but that he had not dared to know it because he was so convinced in his unconscious that any man who hated his mother so intensely without knowing it should not be allowed to love another woman. This, he now declared, was utterly unreasonable.

The final step was postponed for approximately six months and was achieved in the following manner.

Walking down the street, he saw a stranger swearing fluently at a receding car that had splashed water on him. He felt unaccountably impelled to ask the stranger why he was swearing in such a futile fashion. The reply received, as reported by the patient, was, "Oh, it don't do no good, but it makes me feel better and, besides, it wasn't the driver's fault, and my swearing won't hurt him."

The patient related that he became obsessed with this incident for several days before he realized that it constituted an answer to the numerous delays in the execution of many half-formulated plans to stage a quarrel with his mother and "have it out with her." He explained further that an actual quarrel was unnecessary, that a full recognition of his unpleasant emotional attitudes toward his mother, with no denial or repression of them, and in the manner of the man in the street, would permit a true determination of his actual feelings toward his mother. This was the course he followed successfully. By following the example set by the stranger, he successfully established good relationships with his mother.

The remarkable parallelism between this final step and the hypnotic procedure of having him project his experiential life upon hallucinatory figures is at once apparent. It illustrates again the value of the hypnotic utilization of the dynamics of everyday behavior.

COMMENTS

In presenting this case material, the purpose has not been to give an understanding of the dynamics involved in the patient's illness nor of the varied nature of his maladjustments. Rather, the purpose of the entire paper is that of demonstrating the values of hypnotic psychotherapy, methods of application, and technics of utilization. A most important consideration in hypnotherapy lies in the intentional utilization, for corrective purposes, of the mental mechanisms or dynamics of human behavior.

Repressions need not necessarily be broken down by sustained effort. Frequently their maintenance is essential for therapeutic progress. The assumption that the unconscious must be made conscious as rapidly as possible often leads merely to the disorderly mingling of confused, unconscious understandings with conscious confusions and, therefore, a retardation of therapeutic progress.

The dissociation of intellectual content from emotional significances often facilitates an understanding of the meaningfulness of both. Hypnosis permits such dissociation when needed, as well as a correction of it.

Projection, rather than being corrected, can be utilized as a therapeutic activity, as has been illustrated above. Similarly, resistances constituting a part of the problem can be utilized by enhancing them and thereby permitting the patient to discover, under guidance, new ways of behavior favorable to recovery. The tendency to phantasy at the expense of action can be employed through hypnosis to create a need for action.

SUMMARY

In brief, there are three highly important considerations in hypnotic psychotherapy that lend themselves to effective therapeutic results. One is the ease and readiness with which the dynamics and forms of the patient's maladjustments can be utilized effectively to achieve the desired therapy.

Secondly, is the unique opportunity that hypnosis offers to work either separately and independently, or jointly with different aspects of the personality, and thus to establish various nuclei of integration.

Equally important is the value of hypnosis in enabling the patient to re-create and to vivify past experiences free from present conscious influences, and undistorted by his maladjustment, thereby permitting the development of good understandings which lead to therapeutic results.

INDUCED HYPNAGOGIC REVERIES FOR THE RECOVERY OF REPRESSED DATA

BY

LAWRENCE S. KUBIE, M.D.

INTRODUCTION

The hypnagogic reverie might be called a dream without distortion. Its immediate instigator is the day's "unfinished business," but like the dream it derives from more remote "unfinished business" of an entire lifetime as well. The hypnagogic reverie differs from a dream in the fact that there is less elision of the remote and recent past, and far less use of symbolic representation. This would seem to be due to two facts: in the first place, since the reverie does not attempt to say as much as a dream, it does not need to depend upon condensed hieroglyphics to express multiple meanings. In the second place, when the hypnagogic reverie is artificially induced for therapeutic purposes, guilt and anxiety seem to play a less active role than in dreams with the result that the content of the reverie can come through with less disguise. Whatever the explanation, the consequence is that through the induction of states of hypnagogic reverie, significant information about the past can be made readily and directly accessible, without depending upon the interpretations which are requisite in the translation of dreams.

Farber and Fisher[1] have demonstrated that under hypnosis psychologically naïve and uninstructed subjects can translate complex dream symbols without help. Erickson and Kubie[2] have shown that under hypnosis one subject can translate the cryptic automatic writing of another. Perhaps similar mysterious mechanisms make the disguises of dreams less imperative to the hypnagogic reverie than when fully asleep. It is probable that in this partial sleep, in this no-man's land between sleeping and waking, a form of dissociation occurs which makes it possible to by-pass the more obstinate resistances which block our memories in states of full conscious awareness, and which contribute to the distortion of memory traces in dreams.

It is not possible to estimate how widely applicable the hypnagogic reverie may be as a therapeutic technique, nor whether it is useful in certain types of neurotic difficulties and not in others. We cannot say as yet whether it will prove to be useful only when introduced in the course of formal psychoanalytic treatment, or whether it can be used by itself. We can say only that in a number of patients, in whom prolonged analysis had not succeeded in penetrating to the roots of a neurosis, the addition of this technique has proven invaluable. The patient's free associations seem to flow with extraordinary freedom and vividness, gravitating spontaneously to early scenes and experiences with intense affects, yet without the multiple distortions that occur in the dream process. In this way amnestic data have been recovered which proved to be essential to the therapeutic process.

A few earlier workers have been interested in this phenomenon. In 1909 and again in 1911 Silberer[3] reported observations which are tangential to this problem. Sidis[4] in this country was more directly interested in the therapeutic use of this procedure. He induced an hypnoidal state by monotonous reading, singing, and metronome beats, and then asked the subject to "tell what came into his mind . . . during the reading or immediately after." The material that Sidis secured was of considerable interest and had he pursued these observations further and correlated them with the early work of Breuer and Freud and with the developing body of psychoanalytic theory and technique, he would undoubtedly have exercised a profound influence on the development of psychotherapeutic techniques in general.

Two communications have described a simple physiological method for the induction of hypnagogic states (Kubie and Margolin[5, 6]). In this method the subject's own breath sounds are picked up by a contact microphone placed against the neck, amplified, and brought back to the subject through earphones. In most individuals the sound and rhythm of one's own breathing used as a monotonous fixating stimulus has a powerful hypnagogic influence. Difficulties arise occasionally through the occurrence of swallowing noises, coughing, snoring, and the voice sounds themselves, which, because of the amplification, disturb the dozing subject.

Various sedative medications have also been employed, both with and without the breath sound stimulus. Certain of the barbiturates alone, the barbiturates with benzedrine, barbiturates and bromides, and other quite different medications are under investigation.

The hypnagogic reverie has also been induced simply by suggesting total muscular relaxation, much as may be used in the introductory phases of a hypnotic seance, and similar to the procedures recommended by Jacobson.[7] However, the purpose of this report is not to describe technical details of the procedure, but to illustrate from the data of one patient the type of material which can be obtained.

CLINICAL HISTORY

A man in his early forties had been in analysis for a few months in a distant city, when circumstances suddenly forced him to move to New York where, after a short interruption, he continued his analysis with me. He worked at it faithfully and doggedly, but with almost no free associations, no freedom of affect, and few affectively charged memories. In a year and a half of this he had made many secondary symptomatic gains but achieved no deep insight. Then the war intervened to take him to distant regions where there was no possibility of carrying his analytical work further. After an interruption of two years the patient suddenly reappeared in my office in a state of intense inner turmoil and unhappiness. He had taken a leave of absence of less than three weeks in order to attempt to gain some relief. The hypnotic technique described was proposed. The patient was fully aware of the hazardous and uncertain nature of such an undertaking. He was therefore quite ready to cooperate in an attack which both of us regarded as an experiment. In the subsequent two weeks the patient had seventeen sessions. On several occasions he had two sessions in one day, separated by a few hours. Of these seventeen sessions, five were prolonged periods of induced hypnagogic reverie, each lasting from two to four hours. Special time for these was set aside over week-ends, or in the evening. Intervening sessions were of approximately the usual length. The material from these prolonged hypnagogic states will be presented as fully as space permits.

The patient was a young man of exceptional endowments. He had great native intelligence, good education, a privileged position in the community, wealth, physical health, and an attractive appearance. Both parents had been cultured, and socially responsible people of distinction. They had been devoted to each other and to their three children, and had used more than ordinary imagination and feeling in dealing with their children's problems. Nevertheless the patient always felt that he was a fifth wheel to the family wagon, that his father was close to his younger sister and his mother to his older brother, the four of them seeming to him to form an intimate circle from which he was excluded. He had gone through school and college feeling like an unknown, friendless waif. He had pursued a vigorous and not unsuccessful career, yet he felt about it as though it were nothing but a pallid facsimile of his father's life. He had been married twice, but had been unable to accept the rivalry of his own children or of his stepchildren, with the consequence that he had been driven out of both marriages and into hopeless, compulsive promiscuity. Indeed, these transitory relations with women were his only warming intimacies. The pain which these paradoxes and discrepancies cost him was what brought him to analysis.

In every relationship with a woman he was always compelled at first to play the role of the gallant knight saving the lady in distress, only to have the lady in distress turn out to be more boy than girl, a rival rather than a mistress, wholly reluctant to assume the mothering role towards him which he constantly sought.

The acute emotional flurry which occasioned his sudden return to me had been precipitated by a break with just such a woman, which happened to coincide with the sudden collapse of the work to which he had devoted two years of complete absorption. This collapse was occasioned by forces entirely beyond his or anyone else's control, but he had to suffer the added pain of seeing the whole project taken out of his hands and placed in the hands of those who would steer it unwisely and less competently than he.

Although he had been called upon at once to undertake an important new task, he felt unable to launch himself in it. He felt that he could not work and could not stay alone or be with people. He felt physically small, like a shrinking child. He was blue and disheartened. Not ordinarily given to symptomatic anxiety, he found himself restless, jittery and sleepless. His usual imperturbability was broken, and tears were constantly close to the surface. He felt, as he said, "shot" as he had never felt before. It was in this state that we undertook the treatment to be reported.

TREATMENT

The first session was a psychoanalytic hour of the usual type in which the patient reviewed the events leading up to his immediate distress, and described his current symptoms and the ever present sense that rejection was waiting for him.

(1) First Session of Hypnagogic Reverie

The session began at nine in the evening. He reviewed a few of the events of the preceding twenty-four hours, emphasizing particularly the panic that assailed him at the thought of spending the coming holidays alone. Then he was asked to remain silent, listening to his own amplified breath sounds, while focusing his gaze on a small white ring in the center of a large field of grey cloth. He was asked to count his breath sounds silently to himself, "one two, one two" or "in out, in out" (cf. Kubie and Margolin[8]). After ten minutes he was asked. "What has been going on?" and reported that he was concerned chiefly with the mechanics of the apparatus, with ruminations about his tendency to smoke too much, and with his deep conviction that there was something the matter with him.

Again he was asked to be silent, to listen to his breathing as before, and to use his own final question, "What is the matter with me?" as the starting point for his thoughts. I told him I might break in on his silence at any time to ask him what was going on, but that if anything occurred to him that he wanted to communicate to me he should signal to me.

Ten minutes later he signalled and began at once to describe vivid images of himself as a child. Not only was such vivid recall quite absent from his usual associations, but he was able to add certain new items. One was of riding his pony, of jumping it, and falling off, climbing on, jumping it, and again falling off, of doing this over and over although deeply terrified all the while. He was between seven and nine years old when he had this pony. Another memory from the same age period was of persistent nosebleeds. This was linked with a secret fear of all the combative sports in which he took part and led to a memory of wondering whether he was really his parents' child, and to the recovery of a deeply buried rationalization of why he thought that they loved the other two children more than they loved him. "I never had any children's diseases—or did they just not care, and so pretended that I didn't have them?"

This set off another long chain of vivid recollections and images, which will be summarized here as briefly as possible:

It began with mention of his brother's closely-knit, agile, skillful body, in sharp contrast to what he felt to have been his own ungainly size, his fear of boxing, the granulated eyelids he would develop in swimming, his utter terror of diving and inability to dive until he was nearly thirty, his fall from a dam at the age of ten, his father wading in to pull him out, his frantic terror of being clamped down and of having his face smothered under something and of being unable to move his arms, of restricted motion of any kind, the terror he felt at having to crawl under a car to repair anything or to fix tire chains or of putting his head under water, acutely vivid memories of how he felt in the swimming lessons, of squeezing his eyes tight shut and paddling frantically to the edge of the pool, of being terrified to open his eyes until all the water was out. Then came an old, old idea, "it was awful to lose your arms because then you couldn't put your arms around anyone."

It was more important to put your arms around someone than vice-versa. The major bodily injury of his life had been the break which had kept his arm in a cast for months.

This led to a new memory: a bakery cart, the cupcakes from the baker, a secret rendezvous with the baker's cart behind the barn so that the grown-ups wouldn't see. This brought him up against a surprising amnesic gap. He knew that an automobile had been garaged in that barn from the earliest years in which cars were privately owned in this country. He knew that he played in and around that barn-garage from his own earliest years. Yet he had no memory of having seen a car there until years later, nor could he call up an image of any of the horses or carriages in the old barn, nor of the old coachman and his son who was older than the patient. At this point came an image of lying with his face to the ground, among some trees twenty feet from the garage, with the coachman's boy on top of him, his pants down—of being caught there by the governess, and of her promise that she wouldn't tell if he didn't do it again. . . .

At this point the stream ran dry, and he was asked to be silent and to listen quietly to his own amplified breath sounds. About ten minutes later he signalled, and described what he called "odds and ends of ideas." Actually they filled in many details of what had been amnesic a few minutes earlier. There were images of the ground floor in the barn and of the horses themselves, of the end that was reserved for cars when cars first were brought in, of the turnaround back of the stable where there was a tree, marking the place where they met the bakery wagon, of something special about that tree linking it to the coachman's boy whose name he never had been able to recall. There was the business associate whose name he had the embarrassing habit of forgetting and which he now realized was almost identical with the name of this boy. Something was going on between his brother and the coachman's boy. Then came the memory that masturbation began at that time, behind that tree and taught by the coachman's son and by his own older brother. Then he recalled that he had told their tutor what his older brother had taught him, again extracting a promise that the tutor would not tell. He remembered wanting to have both a very large penis and large breasts. He had always taken it for granted that he would have breasts, and he hoped that they would be large. The memory of always telling everything frankly was linked to a feeling that in being frank and open he went too far and got caught, whereas his brother was "cagey" and knew when to stop talking so that he wouldn't get caught.

Then came another memory of a certain kind of naïve remark that he would make, spoken of in the family as a "Tommian remark" (Tommy was not his name but is used for this purpose here). A significant example was that of telling the others that when he brushed his fingernails it made the end of his tongue twitch. He was teased and ridiculed for this; but suddenly he recalled that at a much earlier age he had bitten his nails. To this he added one new bit of historical data: he spoke disparagingly of his unusual ability to think in concrete images as something which was of no consequence at all and of a lifelong conviction that only theoretical abstractions "take brains" and are adult. This led him to an image of his mother reading philosophy aloud to his father, brother and sister, as he sat by, lost in hopeless uncomprehending admiration. He linked this with his first use of a pipe, and his compulsive, excessive pipe smoking.

Against this early ridicule he then set the image of the first occasion on which his father had shown confidence in him. He was in college; his father was very sick, and was dissatisfied with his physician, and wanted to change doctors. He called the patient home and entrusted the arranging of the change to the patient rather than to his older brother or his mother.

After an interval of floundering images came a memory of his mother showing confidence in him. He was nearly twenty. She asked him to help her balance her account. He did this scornfully, making the corrections in bold emphatic figures to indicate his scorn. Then back again to an early memory of Christmas morning, of coming down for their stockings, of finding the stockings filled with coal and kindling but with a five-dollar gold piece in the toe. He could never remember getting his. He was too mad and hurt. This was in no way relieved by the real stocking which came afterward.

Three hours after the session was begun it was interrupted and the patient went home. . . .

(2) *Second Hypnagogic Session*

The next session involving the use of hypnagogic reveries occurred on the following day in the early afternoon. It began with fifteen minutes of silent attention to his amplified breath sounds. At the end of this time he signalled and expressed a desire to describe a "whole series of things that have been going through my mind."

He began by describing his sense of isolation from other boys, his feeling of his inability to do anything as well as they did, and his tendency to console himself and to compensate for this and in a sense to control others through sex. This led to his sense of always overreaching himself, of having gone to college too young, because he had made up three years of preparatory work in a year and a half. He was too young for the S.A.T.C. He was too young when he took over his job. He feels too young now as he faces the new assignment that awaits him. His only compensation is to get a woman under his thumb sexually, so that he can let out his anger, and still save himself from the danger of being alone and from the danger of losing his only potency through masturbation. At this point the thought of waste came to mind and his flow of ideas was blocked. He was again asked to be quiet, to focus his attention on his breath sounds, and to use the concept of waste as the starting point of his reverie.

Ten minutes later he signalled. First there was considerable rumination on the topic of waste and his own general sense of failure. Then he lapsed into silence again, shut his eyes and drifted off for nearly fifteen minutes. Then he signalled again and took up the theme of ridicule and of its relationship to his feeling about the "concrete" and the "abstract," how you couldn't make yourself ridiculous with concrete things whereas it was with regard to "adult abstract things" that he made the old "Tommian remarks," how he was more afraid of ridicule than of anything else in life, and of how the sense of having been ridiculous made him ashamed when at the age of nine he had fallen off a high cross-bar breaking his arm, fracturing his ribs, and dislocating his hip, thus laying himself up for several months. He had been "showing off" to some older boys and girls who were there. It was a high flight followed by a ridiculous fall. It was this that broke his spirit at that time, and not the pain. Then he went on into details of how this feeling had stayed with him, and how it had influenced his relationship to his schoolmates and to his older brother and to all friends.

This was new material and, as he remembered it drowsily, he added further detailed images from his puberty years and early adolescence. Their recital took the rest of the afternoon.

(3) Third Hypnagogic Session

The next afternoon he came for another long session. He went through a short recital of the events of the intervening hours, picking up further ruminations on the general topic of ridicule, his impulse to ridicule others, his incessant sense of being a child vulnerable to the ridicule of grown-ups, and his need to use a woman as someone behind whose skirts he must hide himself or in whose train he might be swept into the company of the mighty.

Then he drifted on into a period of silence, listening quietly to his own breathing, and after about ten minutes, stirred and gave a signal that he wished to communicate something.

It was between the ages of four and five. His father was away. At such times the children in turn were allowed to sleep with their mother, or else just to come in to her bed in the morning. He was sleeping or lying there, cuddling close to her body, feeling how warm and lovely this was. Then suddenly he was being pushed away and was being told that he "was too old for this." He never in his life got into his mother's bed again. He felt guilty, and angry at himself for not having foreseen that this would lose him this warm and glowing opportunity. Once again he had been too "frank and open and direct" instead of sneaking up on it as his brother would have done. Then he thought of a rejected gift that he had bought for a governess, and of feeling ridiculed for wanting to help his teacher by writing sample manuscript letters for her.

After fifteen minutes he lapsed into silence, again focusing on his amplified breath sounds, with his eyes on the white ring—then returned to the critical scene with his mother.

He was lying on his left side. She was lying on her left side. He snuggled up to her that way—"that's the way I always want to go to sleep with a woman even now." The persistent power of the rebuff was so great that he has never held one of his own children in his lap in an affectionate manner, or put his arms around one of them, not with his own nor with any other child. He'd like to do this. (At this point he cried, which was striking in view of the fact that he had never been able to show feelngs in the analysis, nor a moment's tenderness or gentleness to one of his own children or to his stepchildren.)

Suddenly he remembered a later contrasting episode. He was standing next to his mother as the family were playing a game together. Suddenly he found himself with his hand around her waist or shoulder. He felt an intense inner amazement and surprise. He expected momentarily to be pushed away. The surprise was so great that he could not take his mind off of her to think of the game. He kept coming back to her to put his arm around her again. She did not push him away. Then came the thought of his mother and father always very "sweet and affectionate and demon-strative to each other," and of his mother seeming to him to be so towards his brother, and his father towards his sister, but of no one turning towards him.

Then he went back again to the original episode in bed with his mother. He was sure of its sexual nature. It was linked in time with the episode with the coachman's boy. He may have had an erection. He had a vivid kinaesthetic and tactile memory of the sensation all along his body of the area of contact from his chest to his knees as he lay along his mother's lower back, buttocks and thighs.

Then he thought of his mother's words, "you are too old for that," and said he understood for the first time his lifelong and literal fear of growing old. He could remember his belief that parents had intercourse once for each child, which meant that with a family of three or four children intercourse occurred three or four times in a lifetime. Therefore sex and "snuggling" was no part of being an adult and therefore one doesn't want to grow up at all because this meant to lose all hope of what one most wants. Snuggling is a necessary sensation. . . .

After another silence he signalled again, and said "This explains the fascination of breasts. Legs never count, only breasts. . . . As you grow up you come to believe that you should never express any feelings," because whenever he is tired or strained the first thing he wants to do is to cry. He is torn between love of and hate of his mother, between yearning for her and scorn of her. The only feeling he could not hide from himself was rage. If he could only once begin to talk about his feelings he'd "shoot the works." Then came a sudden flood of convincing bits of evidence that his associates in his many activities had great fondness for him; something he had never been able to admit.

Then he suddenly commented "It's funny to have it all bounce up to the present so quickly. It's a funny feeling that the older you get the less possible it gets to express any feelings, and finally even to feel a feeling. Growing up means getting cold and hard and stony, out of terror lest my feelings would run away with me and govern everything. I'm impatient. I wonder about the application of all of this to the problems which face me. . . ."

Suddenly he thought of the fact that every woman he has chosen has always been a woman who is running away from him. Then he said in a rather awed voice, "If mother would ever turn over towards you, then you're as good as father." "To be alone means to be rejected, and what's more to be rejected by mother." "To snuggle up to a woman and go to sleep is more important than intercourse. But mother must be there to let me snuggle. . . ."

These sessions were followed by a series of ordinary psychoanalytic sessions, interspersed with two shorter sessions of hypnagogic states. These evoked no new material but reworked the data that had already been covered, relating them in many different ways to the problems which had beset the patient all through his life. He became increasingly eager to return to his job and actually cut short his holiday to do so. He saw the woman who had been concerned in the precipitation of the acute illness and had a feeling, as he put it, that he "could take her or leave her" without its being a catastrophe either way, and that he "saw her as a human being" for the first time. He felt physically as large as anyone in his office, instead of feeling physically "overawed and little," in a world of towering rooms and furnishings and giants. His feeling of his own body seemed suddenly to mature (it should be borne in mind that this was a man of more than average size, broad shouldered, and athletic).

His own subjective impression was that the long hypnagogic reveries seemed to bring up not only the new factual data, but all of the attendant sensations and affects which linked them dynamically with his life.

It is unfortunate that the written records of these events can give so little of the breath of life which infused the memories themselves. For this reason, however, it is impossible adequately to convey the contrast between the barren sterile intellectuality of the preceding years of analysis, and the free affectivity of the memories recaptured and revivified in these hypnagogic reveries.

In a peaceful and optimistic state he returned to work. Eight months later he reported that he has been steadier, more cheerful, and more independent than ever before in his life.

With a patient who had been in analysis for a long time, it is impossible to say that the months of analytical work did not in some measure color, or provide material for the data obtained subsequently in hypnagogic reveries. We can say only that in this particular patient the material had remained inaccessible until this technique was added. The degree to which similar material is accessible by this technique in patients who have not been in analysis, will have to be demonstrated in later communications. At this point we can say only that we have had enough experience with the method with patients who have not been analyzed to feel that the same basic forces are at work in both groups, and that the recovery of buried amnestic data is greatly facilitated by the use of hypnagogic reveries irrespective of analysis.

HYPNOTIC RELAXATION
AND ANALYSIS

BY

JACOB H. CONN, M.D.

Modern psychiatry began when the patient was given an opportunity to participate in his own treatment. To the concept of psychotherapy as being primarily *patient-centered* has been added the fundamental clinical observation that the patient can objectively experience what he is doing and, for the first time, bring together the motives of his behavior in a controlled interpersonal relationship. This dynamic experience of the patient knowing, accepting and realizing himself as a unique individual, at first in a therapeutic milieu and later under actual living conditions, has been the goal of every type of psychotherapy, with the exception of hypnotherapy, in recent years.

When the astrological and ceremonious trappings of Mesmer (1734–1815) were finally displaced by the vague concept of suggestion as formulated by Bernheim (1837–1919), the victory, as far as the patient was concerned, was only a nominal one. The practice of hypnotism continued along two established directions— the "suggested" disappearance of symptoms either by command or by recall of a specific traumatic situation with its associated "emotional" catharsis.

During the past few decades a growing emphasis has been placed upon meeting the specific psychologic needs of the patient in the trance state and the necessity for making the interpersonal situation as effective as possible. Erickson, who probably is the most ingenious and clinically astute hypnotist of our time, repeatedly has stressed "the great need for the patient to participate actively in any reorganization of his psychic life," and has advised that "the hypnotist should use that technique which permits him to express himself most satisfactorily and effectively in the special interpersonal relationship which constitutes hypnosis."

Brenman and Gill, in their excellent review of hypnotherapy, have restated Schilder's shrewd observation that "there is no necessary relation between the depth of hypnosis, as the concept is ordinarily understood, and the depth of hypnosis in the sense of the extent to which the individual's personality is really involved in the hypnotic state." One individual in the somnambulist stage may be essentially little involved in the hypnotic state, whereas another individual in a light state of hypnosis may be deeply involved. Erickson's experiences also corroborate this significant clinical observation. Thus he points out that "the phenomena usually found in deep hypnosis may, in the individual subject, occur in light hypnosis and vice versa, depending upon the subject's personality and his psychological needs at the time."

The author has found that light hypnotic trance, induced without specific sleep suggestions, facilitates the recall and analysis of repressed material. Like other hypnotic techniques, this one results in a substantial reduction of the time which would otherwise be required if free association alone were employed. This method has the overall advantage that it is adaptable to patients who may not be amenable to the usual type of hypnotic trance induction.

THE INDUCTION OF THE TRANCE STATE

After the spontaneous complaint-problem, the pertinent historical setting and the development of the present illness have been learned, and a satisfactory patient-physician relationship is intuitively felt to be present, a brief discussion of the value of "relaxation" as contrasted to the previous "tension" state is introduced in a matter-of-fact manner. The patient then is requested to get up from the office chair and to sit in a more comfortable armchair in order to become "more relaxed." Not infrequently brief mention is made of the "wonderful work" which is being done by the psychiatrists in the Armed Forces in "curing" their patients with this same method of relaxation. The patient is asked to make himself comfortable and to look up at a bright object which is placed several inches from his eyes and just above the horizontal line of vision (after Braid and Bernheim).

The author *carefully defines how he expects the patient to act* saying, "You will *not* fall asleep, so that we can talk things over when you are completely relaxed. The muscles of your legs and arms are becoming more relaxed, the muscles of your stomach, chest and neck are relaxed. Your facial muscles are relaxed. Your eye muscles are relaxed. They are beginning to close. They are closing. You are going into a deep, natural relaxed state." At this point the object in the physician's hand is slowly lowered and the patient usually follows it with his eyes until the lids are almost closed and begin to flicker. The physician then continues to lower the object in his hand until it is below the line of vision and then quietly says, "Your eyes are closed." In some cases the result is a continuous fluttering of the closed lids which causes the patient to remark, "What is the matter with my eyes?" In other individuals the eyes remain open and staring until the direction, "shut your eyes," is given. The entire procedure takes about three to five minutes.

The patient now is resting quietly and "exhibiting the air of abstraction" and drowsiness, the decrease of initiative and spontaneity, the relative lack of humor and self-consciousness which usually are found in the altered state known as hypnosis (Wells). Following a brief period of silence, the doctor says: "Just enjoy being relaxed. Enjoy being your real self. If anything comes to your mind and you feel like talking about it, do so, but let it come without straining, without any effort on your part to please me. Let it come as easily as breathing." The patient is then directed to "breathe in" and "breathe out" in a rhythmic manner thus keeping him "listening" and close to the waking state.

After several more minutes have elapsed the patient is asked, "What comes to your mind?" The usual response is "Nothing." This is only partly indicative of the lack of spontaneity induced by the trance state; it also is due to the *need for further direction*. The patient is waiting for clues and hints as to how to behave and what to look for in order to please the hypnotist-physician.

As will repeatedly be demonstrated, the patient has been trying to please everyone about him for many years in a desperate effort to lose himself and his individuality. This concept has been described in detail by Erich Fromm, who quotes the following from Dostoevski's "The Brothers Karamasov": "He has no more pressing need than the one to find someone to whom he can surrender, as quickly as possible, that gift of freedom which he, the unfortunate creature, was born with." Fromm continues, "The frightened individual seeks for somebody or something to tie his self to; he cannot bear to be his own individual self any longer, and he tries frantically to get rid of it and to feel security again by the elimination of this burden: the self."

In keeping with these observations, the doctor replies to the patient, who has stated that "nothing" is on his mind, as follows: "Enjoy being fully relaxed. You have nothing on your mind; that is good. Don't say anything until it comes to you naturally and without effort. What you say is not as important as how you act in keeping with your natural, real feelings. You can say nothing and get well if that is what you want to do."

When lid catalepsy is not produced by the above procedure, the question is asked, "What seems to be the matter?" and an attempt is made to remove the "resistance"; then the procedure is begun all over again. It is seldom necessary to repeat it more than three times. If the third attempt fails, the author says, "You are not ready to be relaxed. You still are too tense. This can be done later when you are more at ease," or "We don't have to do it this way. We are working out a method which is best suited to *you* and to *your* specific problems. If this method works it should work without any effort; it should be *exactly* what *you* need and what you can enjoy doing, otherwise we will find a more suitable method of treatment for your particular case."

An example of a "failure" which was turned into a "success" is that of a 30-year-old immature married woman who no longer was on speaking terms with her mother whom she "accused" of favoring another sibling. The patient did not respond to the first two attempts to induce a trance state. When asked what seemed to be the trouble, she replied, "I don't want to be a marionette. About a year ago I told you I dreamed that I was a marionette. I have been telling you how my mother would push me around. I feel the same way now." ("Am I pushing you around? Aren't you doing this to help yourself?") "I realize you are not pushing me around but that's the way I feel about it." ("Then let's try it again.") The patient closed her eyes and went into the trance state soon after the next few words were spoken.

THE USE OF THE TRANCE STATE
AS AN INTEGRATED EXPERIENCE

(CASE STUDIES)

The method as outlined above can be utilized not only to elicit content, but as a creative, dynamic experience in which the patient may develop a more adequate realization of what self-acceptance actually means.

The author makes it a rule never to "challenge" the patient to try to open his eyes nor does he attempt to test the "depth" of the trance state. The patient soon begins to realize that the total treatment program is oriented in the direction of self-acceptance.

The awareness of self as an actuality may be realized in its proper perspective in the hypnotic state. The contrast between just "talking things over" and the impact of reality as a vital experience is illustrated by the next case.

Samuel C., age 43, had been involved in an obsessive-compulsive ruminative tension state for 30 years. He had developed a syphilophobia and numerous obsessive compulsive rituals. During a series of hypnotic sessions he was able for the first time to experience a sense of integrated subject organization which helped him to resolve his chronic state of self-doubt and accept himself for what he really was—an immature individual who had thought of himself as living in a world of threatening adults. For fifteen years the patient had been "terrified" following a flirtation with a married woman whose husband had threatened to thrash him if he ever did it again. Since then Mr. C. had obsessively watched what went into and what came out of every pocket and dreaded to send his clothes to the cleaners for fear that a piece of paper bearing his address might fall out.

During the trance state the patient felt "relaxed" for the first time in many years and stated, "I was afraid to let one thought interfere with another; even thinking of other things might throw me off guard. . . . Whenever I saw a girl I turned my head. . . . I was afraid it (sex) would excite me too much. I was almost jarred when I found out I wasn't fighting anything. I was terribly surprised that when (since the previous session) I looked at a girl two or three times that the desire disappeared. I had the idea that the more I looked at girls the more I would want to. It turned out to be just the opposite. I was constantly fooling myself. I never trusted myself. . . . There is no sense in fighting myself. . . . Suppose something does fall out of my pockets. Suppose my name and address do fall out. Gee Zu! that was 15 years ago. To remember for 15 years what a man said in 15 seconds! I must of been frightfully frightened at the time." (The patient was taken out of the trance state and asked, "Why didn't you see all this before?") "I would sit there confused and paralyzed by fear and would not be able to digest the words. We'd be discussing why I would worry over the piece of paper or how I closed a door. We never got to the point where I could calm myself down. As I got myself to relax I could see that those terrific fears were no longer fears. I would hear you say that what I was doing was not normal but I wouldn't believe it. With this (hypnosis) it meant something. I absorbed the words; they became part of me."

The confronting of the experiencing portion of the self with that part of the personality which has been excluded from consciousness is well illustrated in the next patient.

Charles S., age 27, had been a timid child who had become fearful in the first grade; he had developed an acute anxiety state at the age of 18 during a vacation trip, and became increasingly apprehensive about being trapped in "closed spaces." His claustrophobia became acute in 1940, causing him to terminate his professional studies. His lack of self-assertion ("I can't argue. I walk away.") and pathologic self-consciousness ("I feel everyone is looking at me") finally brought him for treatment.

The patient had been under treatment several months when he

reported a dream saying, "I wonder why I dream the same thing again and again. I see a man in a dark cape and black hat. He just stands there and glares in the dark." The patient went into the trance state before the words, "You will become completely relaxed," were said.

("You can see that man now.") "I see that fellow with the cape standing under a tree. He is standing there waiting for me to do something. It seems I was the one who did the running; he never ran after me. I'd run from him." ("From whom?") "I am not sure but he looks something like me. I was trying to run away from myself. He looked awfully angry. I never associated the dreams with the way I felt. Now I can see it. I was runnig away from the part I am afraid of, the bad part." ("What part?") "The part that acts like a man, like a tough man." ("Now you feel?") "That I can say what I think and what I feel." ("Why?") "I have been afraid to be myself. I didn't know that I was afraid to be myself. I thought I was myself." ("Why should you have had this dream at this time?") "There is always something at home (where he lives with his domineering. neurotic mother) that makes me angry. Something happened and I kept it back. I didn't say anything, I wasn't true to myself."

Psychoanalytic literature contains many references to one of the most difficult obstacles to therapeutic success, namely, the male patient's rejection of his passive homosexual femininity. The next patient demonstrates how this problem was handled by hypnotic relaxation and analysis.

Robert N., age 23, was referred for psychiatric treatment shortly after being discharged from the armed services because of a "severe psychoneurosis." He stated that he was afraid to leave his house and was "very self-conscious." He recalled being fearful of other children since the age of eight because they would beat him and call him "fatty." After graduating from college he entered a professional school where he developed "nervous headaches," became too upset to complete his freshman examinations and was asked to leave. He then was drafted, and found himself unable to adjust to military life. He recalled feeling "small and inconspicuous" in his uniform and how he had felt "overdressed and too conspicuous" in civilian clothes. Mr. N. gradually became more upset by military routine, found that he "couldn't take orders" from those whom he considered to be his "inferiors with sixth-grade educations," and "burned up" that he had not been able to "rate a commission." After six months in military service he was discharged with a diagnosis of "anxiety-neurosis." For several years the patient had experienced a compulsion to make certain that he was dressed "perfectly" before leaving the house, had developed a strong feeling that people were observing him whenever he rode on streetcars so that he felt compelled to ride only in taxicabs.

The hypnotic interviews took place twice weekly. The patient was readily hypnotized. He spontaneously stated that he had been greatly concerned because he had "a very small penis," and that this "fact" had been a source of marked inferiority feelings. The patient also spoke of preferring "older, buxom women" to girls of his own age, and added that, "Even when the woman says that she is satisfied with me as a sexual partner, I feel that she doing me a favor." All of his sex experiences had been with "cheap" prostitutes as he had never been at ease with girls of his own educational and social status. Mr. N. also referred to his ambition either to become a doctor or an author of short stories.

During the second hypnotic interview the patient mentioned that he had been "terribly embarrassed" by frequent blushing and a compulsion to avert his eyes since the age of 13. He recalled that his mother had "caught" him masturbating and had sternly admonished him "never to do such a horrible thing again." Mr. N. said, "I kept on doing it but I always felt I would be found out. When my mother looked at me, I felt she might read my thoughts, so I tried to hide them by averting my eyes. . . . I even thought of my sister doing the same thing. It made me ashamed." The patient went on to describe how "insignificant and small" he had felt and that he had worn padded clothes for the past four years. He said, "I was always wondering if others could see my feminine characteristics. I haven't gone swimming for years because of my flabby skin and small shoulders. It's all related to having a small penis. I even feel like describing a beautiful scene in poetic language—like a woman does." ("Suppose it is like a woman—what is wrong about that—why can't you be—?") "Myself." ("You always have to be?") "Like someone else." ("The point is?") "To be myself. The hell with the attitudes of other people towards me. When I was fat (age eight) I thought people were going to laugh at me. I still picture myself as being a very chubby, white-skinned kid with a protruding belly and a shriveled penis. I masturbated with the idea that the penis would stretch and grow. When I was about 12 (while swimming) I saw my father's penis; his was small compared to other men. I take after my father, a small, undignified man with no great future ahead of him. My mother runs the show. She brought me up with the idea that I was going to be a top man—a doctor, since it meant prestige and money. It all went against the grain." ("Then you were a legitimate failure in professional school?") "We are always getting back to myself." ("You were scared to be anything but what your mother expected you to be.") "I was afraid to hurt her, she is so emotional and high-strung. I felt I had to be looked up to so I had to look very presentable. I had to be perfect sexually and I had to be a dominating personality." ("But that's not really you.") "I was the person my mother was trying to make me. I was my mother." ("Now you can say, 'I will be myself. I will trust my real feelings, my real self.' ") (Repeats) "It is a tremendous relief for me to say that; I was afraid of being dominated by my mother, like my poor father." ("Now you can understand why you blushed?") "It's feminine; it's like the idea of having a small penis. I can see that it's dangerous to become what my mother wants me to become."

The patient stated that he never really had wanted to enter a profession or to write for a living. He now had an opportunity to learn the insurance business and felt that this was what he wanted as it was his own decision.

During the ninth hypnotic session (May 27) he stated, "My fears in life were silly, nonsensical. I just didn't have a backbone because I was dominated." ("Were you *really?*") "No. I allowed my mother to dominate me. I *wanted her to;* my mother is selfish and makes my father cry. I can see in him a mirror image of myself. I feel I realize what my mother has tried to do with me." ("That's called being grown up.") "I was a kid before. I blushed like a woman—like my mother."

On June 9 (tenth hypnotic session) the patient reported, "My mother doesn't worry me any more. I used to dread telling her what time I'd be home. Now I come and go as I please. I just don't answer her if she gets upset."

The patient also had been taking out a "nice" girl for the first time. He said, "I felt wonderful. It's doing something that I've always wanted to do but was afraid to do, because of my fear of blushing and my worry over having a small penis."

He again discussed a recent sex experience saying, "I find sex actually enjoyable, not in the sense of building up my ego. I found it nice relaxation." ("Before?") "It was making myself what I really wasn't, a man. I used to ask each woman in a round about way, 'Did I satisfy you?' They'd say, 'Yes'; no woman ever told me, 'No,' and yet I'd walk out in doubt." ("Who insisted on that?") "I did. I insisted on being in doubt. I wanted to insist on it. I didn't want to be a man. I wanted to be a replica of my mother so I insisted that I had a small penis." ("Why?") "So that I wouldn't have the responsibility of being myself." ("If you were like her?") "It would put me in the exact path my mother wanted me to go. Normal sex would take me away from those paths. My mother said sex was wrong, that it would ruin me." ("And the blushing?") "I felt I was a woman. At home with my mother and (13-year-old) sister, I'd feel a blush coming up when I'd realize that I was talking like a woman, like one of them. With one of my friends I'd feel self-conscious as if he were looking at me, as if he thought I was a woman when I'd say something in a feminine way. I insisted on being recognized as being a woman and then blamed it on others!"

On July 8 the patient reported having gone swimming for the first time in four years and of feeling comfortable on the beach. The last (14th session) took place on July 22, 1945.

The hypnotic interviews had taken place over a period of five months (March–July). A follow-up visit two years later (June 6) included a report of being free of his former neurotic complaints and that the patient was well adjusted at work and at home.

The following two cases illustrate the use of hypnotic relaxation and analysis of convicted sex offenders whose sentences were suspended with the understanding that they would accept psychiatric treatment during the period of probation. They were referred to the author by the Supreme Bench of Baltimore, acting upon the recommendation of its Chief Medical Officer, Dr. Manfred S. Guttmacher. [Incidentally, in his recent book, "Sex Offenses," Dr. Guttmacher has stated, "Probably the most extensive series of sex offenders treated psychotherapeutically, and also the series in which the best results are reported achieved, is that of Dr. Jacob H. Conn, published in The Journal of Clinical Psychopathology in 1949."][1]

Mr. C., age 31, presented a serious dilemna to both the Judge and the court psychiatrist. The parents of the girl who had been forced to practice fellatio were adamant in their insistence that the patient be "put behind bars." They repeatedly stated that he should receive a sentence longer than ten years since another sex offender who recently had been involved with an older child had received a ten-year sentence. The parents were convinced that the child's complaint of abdominal distress which recurred every few days was the result of having swallowed semen, but they refused to permit the Chief Medical Officer to arrange to have the child examined by a psychiatrist. The father vehemently objected to any possible treatment plan for the patient and emphatically denied that he "hated any man." As evidence of his good will he volunteered to go to the penitentiary every day and pray with the patient "so that God would enter his heart." The police report included the fact that the patient had picked up two children, ages 7 and 6, and had shown them nude pictures, had exposed himself, had given a knife to the older child and told her to "cut it off." He then shoved her head down and put his penis in her mouth and ejaculated. This ejaculation into the child's mouth was denied by the patient. After this incident he had returned the two children to the school where he had picked them up.

Mr. C. was properly identified. The book with the nude pictures and the knife were found in his car. Nevertheless he continued to deny that he was the man involved in the offense. The court psychiatrist talked with him of the futility of psychiatric treatment unless he was going to be honest in admitting and facing his problems. The only alternative to accepting treatment being a long period of incarceration, the patient admitted the offense and began to relate his "profound neurotic problems." Mr. C. began treatment on May 16, 1947, with the statement: "I just cannot control my sexual emotions. I don't get too much intercourse, only two or three times a week. Then I jerk off two and sometimes as much as four times a day. I also have wet dreams two or three times a week" (for the past four years). The patient stated that this was the first time that he had used a child as a sexual object and readily admitted that he had requested the older girl "to bite" his penis or "to cut it off." He went on to describe his severe anxiety state which began in 1943 and included bouts of diarrhea, sweating and attacks of palpitation, terrifying dreams of being in a car rolling down the hill out of control, or dreams of being chased by wild animals while hunting and finding that his gun "won't work." Because of the anxiety and pathologic tension, the treatment selected in this case was *hypnotic relaxation* and the fostering of a sense of freedom to talk or to keep silent if he so preferred. The aim was to have him feel comfortable in the therapist's presence and he was repeatedly instructed during the hypnotic interview not to say anything unless he could do so without effort.

The result of the treatment has been a realization of the patient's previous passive dependent sexual character and a growing ability to accept a normal heterosexual role. Thus he could say: "It never dawned on me before that this girl (his boyhood sweetheart) used to put it in her mouth for me." He recalled that he had pushed the child's mouth on his penis, then had masturbated after she had left the car. The patient said, "I thought then of the girl back home putting it in her mouth; that proved she really cared for me. She was hot natured and from a fine family. She did this so we wouldn't have intercourse. I guess it satisfied her desires too." He has had psoriasis since he was two years old, and had thought of himself as being a freak. He said, "I just didn't know anyone else who had this skin condition except my three first (maternal) cousins. I never could go in swimming or go in for athletics in high school or college. I was ashamed to undress before anyone. I felt no one could care for me. I knew this girl liked me so I hung on to her."

As the weekly interviews continued Mr. C. was surprised to learn that he wasn't as "hot natured" as he thought he was. The patient, who had believed that he was a sexual athlete because of his orgiastic frequency, began to experience satisfying sexual relief when he began having heterosexual marital relations twice a week. The important clue to his sexual tension was the fact that he had been apprehensive about losing his girl friend. He feared that he might never find another, and had built up an idealized image of her. He had thought of himself as being over-sexed because of that "over-charged feeling" and stated, "The only way to get rid of it was to jerk off." Mr. C. began to understand the manner in which he had increased his sex tension. He said, "I always carried a picture of this girl in my mind. I always was thinking of her and her big breasts." In 1941 (age 24) he had married an attractive young woman but had continued to daydream about his idealized former sex partner. During the third hypnotic session (May 2, 1947) Mr. C. spoke of her beauty. He was told to take a good look at her when he visited his parents who lived in the same town. The patient returned with the following account. "You told me to talk to her and to see her as she really was. I never had taken a good look. I never had compared her with my wife. When I saw her as she was, there was no comparison (with my wife.) She had put on weight and was all out of shape. I had carried in my mind that this girl was something like a goddess, real beautiful. I had seen her before (on previous visits to his home) but it didn't soak in. I had always carried in my mind the picture of how she used to be. When I saw her as she really was I could forget her." He had begun a masturbatory and fellatio relationship with this girl when he was 15 years of age (1932) and had continued it until he was 23 (1940). He would have continued this relationship but the girl suddenly stopped seeing him without offering him an excuse. The patient had married his wife on the rebound five months after being jilted. He then found himself restricted to two or three intercourses a week and with no outlet for his compulsive passive-dependent sexual needs. During the war years he also became increasingly upset by the threat of being drafted and very concerned whether or not he should buy a house. Mr. C. rationalized his mounting tension as being due to his fear of further contributing to his mother's distress if he were drafted, as his younger brother already was in the service. In this setting of an idealized image of a boyhood sex partner, situational stress and anxiety derived from frustrated passive-dependent sexual needs, his tension mounted, overflowing into the cardiovascular, muscular, gastrointestinal and sexual systems.

The patient who was first interviewed on May 16, 1947, could report ten weeks later on September 2 that most of his anxiety manifestations had disappeared. He was sleeping soundly and his previous marked sex tension had been reduced to normal. The fearful dream contents were no longer present, being replaced by pleasant dream experiences. He began putting on weight and has gained from 170 to 197 pounds during the first six months of treatment (May, 1947 to November, 1947). He repeatedly spoke of being more at ease than he had been for many years. He ascribed the greatest effect of the treatment, first, to the shattering of the idealized image of his boyhood sweetheart; second, to learning that he was not different from others (a "freak") because of his skin disease, psoriasis; and, third, to the hypnotic relaxation. He recently stated: "You told me (during a hypnotic interview on May 27) that Helen (the previous sex partner) was no good for me (because she had fostered the patient's passive-dependent tendencies). I saw her on June 2, 1947. (Psychiatric treatment had begun on May 16.) She looked like she had been through the mill. Her face was broken out, her color bad. She was fat. I never did care for fat women. Before I felt I never could get well. I felt out of place and kept to myself. I found out I wasn't the only one who had psoriasis. I got all this off of my chest. I began to feel I was like a lot of others. I had thought I had a blood disease so what was the use if it all came from the inside. When you said this disease (psoriasis) occurs in the healthiest people it made me feel good." The patient had been instructed to bring in a weekly report. On January 6, 1948 (seven months after the initial visit), he wrote, "I sleep good, eat good and feel good. No more dreams about women and sex. Boy, am I glad!" On June 6, 1948, he reported, "I never felt better in my life."

One more item should be presented. For the first time since his psoriasis had appeared at the age of 3 the patient was free of lesions for a two-year period. Mr. C. had been given repeated hypnotic suggestions (since August, 1947) to think that his skin would be clear, and was told, "Since you have become so different, so will your skin," or "Your gain in weight is a proof of the change. Every spot that was 'sick' will become well." Since childhood the patient's psoriasis had reappeared each year by October 1. Now for the first time in 28 years he did not develop psoriatic lesions.

In November, 1948, the patient reported that he was experiencing satisfactory marital sex relations once or twice a week. The fatigue and anxiety state which had been present since 1942 had disappeared. Mr. C. was interviewed (during hypnosis) weekly for a period of a year (1947); then every two weeks for four months and every three weeks thereafter, September, 1948 to March, 1949. He had maintained his progress when interviewed on March 11, 1949. During these two years (1947–1949) the patient has been gainfully employed. During the last interview he stated, "If anyone would have told me that it was possible to feel as I do now a year ago, I would have said that he was crazy."

Mr. D., age 32, was described as a model husband, a devoted father and a good neighbor. His daughter had been operated on for a brain tumor when she was 11 months old in 1946 and had died in May, 1948. His wife had become depressed and their sex relations became infrequent and unsatisfying. In May, 1947, the patient saw two 12-year-old girls dancing in a school yard and exposed himself. He was arrested, released on collateral and did not return to court. Mr. D. later was warned by a park policeman after taking several children for a ride and again was arrested in August, 1948 by the same officer for engaging in lewd and obscene conversation with children. The sentence was suspended, and the patient was referred for psychiatric treatment on September 25, 1948.

The patient began the first interview (he was seen once a week) by saying, "The children had deliberately attracted my attention. They were pleased when I did it and acted forward and wanted me to act forward. I always was obliging, so I obliged." While in a hypnotic trance on November 14, 1948, he was able to say, "I wanted to do something different. Something I had never done before. I just wanted to do something for myself, to relieve myself. Before, I had done things to please other people; this time I was going to please myself. It feels pretty good to say that." During the next hypnotic interview (November 21) he continued, "Now I can say that I did something for myself. I really learned that lesson here." (The patient referred to the repeated suggestion that he take care of himself and not try to please the therapist or anyone else. During a previous session he had refused to permit another patient to precede him into the office by asserting that the appointment was his, and he was complimented for taking care of himself. The patient was now ready to reveal to himself the pattern of neurotic compliance which had been present for many years.) Mr. D. continued, "I never did anything for myself before I showed myself to those girls. I would always accede to anybody's request. They didn't have to command me, even before they'd ask me I would do it. I didn't even think I was pleasing them. I'd think I was pleasing myself by being a nice guy."

The patient had been married twice. During his first marriage at age 16 he had been informed by his wife that a man had exposed himself to her in a public library. He recalled (while in the trance state) that he had thought of the exposure not as being wrong but as an act during which the man had "boldly satisfied himself." He added, "It was something to look up to rather than to punish. I felt all those years that I too should be satisfying myself. Lots of times I should have said 'No' rather than 'Yes' to those who asked a favor, but I never did it." He said, "When I ever had any forwardness presented to me by a woman I thought I had to go the whole way or do nothing. That's why when a married woman sat on my lap at a party I never hugged her. I always thought I had to go the whole way to please a woman even if she exposed her leg. Now I realize that they are kidding or having fun. I am starting to realize (at age 32) that women can do these things and not expect me to give in to them . . . I was always serious and when I started something I'd finish it. I thought all women were that way. I always dreaded that they might say, 'No' so I never asked for anything of anyone." A week later (November 28, during the 10th hypnotic interview) he could say, "I just let myself believe the children were asking me to expose myself. I was pleasing myself. I seem to be growing up. I did what I always had refrained from doing—pleasing myself."

This patient had never had the usual sex experiences of childhood. He recalled, "I can see that I actually missed a lot. I never went through a period of masturbation (or peeping or childhood exhibitionism). I started going with my first wife at 14, had intercourse with her and married her (at age 16) when she became pregnant. I didn't know that she had been secretly married and running around (promiscuous)." This marriage broke up two years later when the patient was 18 years old. This data makes possible another formulation than that which is usually offered in the literature. Instead of always positing a regression to less complex, outmoded but previously satisfying sex patterns, this patient's exhibitionism represents a progression. He is starting to grow and is becoming an active agent by unconsciously asserting himself as he should have done 25 years previously. Mr. D. is correct when he says, "I seem to be growing up." He now can discuss the genesis of his passive-dependent needs. His younger brother had been the mother's favorite. The patient had taken over the responsibility of watching over him in an overly conscientious manner. On several occasions when the brother was almost killed the patient developed intense feelings of guilt although he had done all he could to prevent these near fatal accidents. After this material was reviewed he asked, "Could it have been that by losing my brother I would have been able to live my own life? I wouldn't let myself believe that I could do without him. It never occurred to me if he were not with me I could do other things."

On March 20 (24th session) the patient brought together his compulsive need to watch over his younger brother, his desire to please his parents in order to gain acceptance, and his masochistic need to surrender his independence. He summed up this insight by saying, "If my brother had been killed, I would have found my fears false. I really wasn't responsible for my brother, but then I would have learned to live for myself. I wouldn't take a chance of testing this, that is, putting my parents' love for me to a test. I was afraid the answer would be 'no.' " On March 27 (27th session) he reported that he had gained fourteen pounds, and that he was feeling "like a different person." He said, "I think of other people differently. I am growing up mentally and sexually. Now I don't pay any attention to it when women stand close to me." (Before?) "I always moved away." (Why?) "It was a fear of being censured." Mr. D. recalled the episode of exposure and explained it by saying,

"I wanted to be entirely different than I ever was before. I thought that they (the girls) would do the same (exhibit themselves). I had never seen any girl's privates. A boy (at age 10) once told me that as girls grew older their openings grew. I didn't believe it. I wanted to satisfy myself whether I was right or wrong. I remember he got mad with me because I didn't agree with him." At a recent party the patient had kissed a woman while dancing with her and was not rebuffed. During the following interview (April 3) he said, "If only you had talked to me when I was 14. I just felt a fear of censure all of these years. When a woman refused to dance with me, I asked her why. She said her feet hurt. (Previously) I never made an effort to find out why. I would blame myself. I always blamed myself, and I bought security. I had no desire to be big. I always wanted to stay little. I even thought when I grew up tall like my father I would fall over. I didn't want to grow up. I was upset when my parents quarrelled; I didn't want to go through that. I didn't want to grow up. I was afraid to take care of myself. I took care of my brother so I wouldn't have my own self to worry about."

At the end of the six-month period of treatment (September, 1948 to April, 1949) the patient was asserting himself normally at work, at home and socially. ("I am more forceful. I speak out. Before, I'd give in even when I knew that I was right.") When last interviewed on August 5, 1951 he was happier, able to think and act in keeping with his actual needs, well adjusted sexually and free from the compulsive urge to exhibit himself.

CONCLUSIONS

Psychotherapy has developed into a dynamic interpersonal experience. The traditional concept of hypnosis as being a passive, physician-centered technique is no longer in accord with accepted psychologic theory and the facts derived from clinical practice. The newer conceptions of hypnosis have contributed to its utilization for a more active, patient-centered therapy.

The clinical material which has been presented would indicate that the patients who never have been able to assert themselves,

who are always self-effacing and looking for cues and hints as to
how to please others, will tend to behave in the same manner
during the hypnotic situation.

Hypnosis is an altered psychologic state, a particular type of
behavior which is closer to the waking state than to physiologic
sleep. It can be utilized therapeutically for active patient-partici-
pation as a creative, unifying interpersonal experience and therefore can be classified as a form of dynamic psychotherapy.

HYPNOANALYSIS

BY

ROBERT M. LINDNER, Ph.D.

Hypnoanalysis is a radically abbreviated form of deep psychotherapy which takes its departure from psychoanalysis but which confirms rather than disputes the findings of the more orthodox analytic approach.

Hypnoanalysis is a term properly reserved for those therapeutic efforts in which hypnosis is combined with the techniques of psychoanalysis in service of the goals of treatment. That is to say, the propositions basic to hypnoanalysis are derived from dynamic depth psychology, and the methodological approach incorporates hypnosis. The exact ingredients of this combination depend upon the variant of hypnoanalysis employed. The one which will concern us here is the variant which I have shared in developing, but the aims of all forms of hypnoanalysis are similar. They are: (a) to seek out the hidden pathogenic agents; (b) to realize an abreaction in which the total personality shares; and (c) to more hygienically redistribute the energies formerly exploited by the pathological processes.

In the variant of hypnoanalysis with which I am best acquainted, intensive training in hypnosis marks the opening phase of treatment. Patients are instructed in hypnosis, their misconceptions regarding it are dispelled, they are literally *taught* how to be hypnotized. The extent of the period of training is approximately one week. During the daily session, the special problem or perplexity which encouraged the patient to seek help is not discussed. At the end of this initial period, the patient should possess three capabilities which are necessary to the progress of the analysis: he should be able to enter the trance state immediately upon the suggestion of the hypno-analyst; he should be able to carry out post-hypnotic suggestions with ease and rapidity; he should be able to revert memorially to former scenes and places. This latter capability presents a delicate problem, calling for the exercise of considerable care. The clinician must encourage two varieties of memorial reversion: the *regressive*—where the patient recalls previous experiences but views them in the light of his present outlook—and the *revivified*—where the patient actually relives the event by returning to the previous biographical setting and literally participating in it once more.

The second phase of therapy utilizes the method of free-association. The patient is directed to choose a starting point and to associate without regard to form or content. The usual psychoanalytic principles are followed as hour succeeds hour. When resistances are encountered, however, free-association is abandoned for hypnotic recall. Resistances are not analyzed, but rather undercut. The patient is hypnotized and urged to reveal the nature of the matter to which he has demonstrated reluctance. If the matter is biographical, either regression or revivification may be employed, although it appears preferable to call upon the former in early phases of treatment and the latter later on. The so-called *interim phenomenon* enters at this point. Research has revealed that an unvarying sequence of events transpire when hypnotic recall is performed in the course of an hypnoanalysis: (1) resistance to free-association is present: (2) the patient recounts or reenacts the crucial material, be it event or phantasy; (3) soon thereafter the same material to which resistance had formerly been shown, if it is memorially valid, appears in the waking state in free-association. What apparently takes place to account for this important phenomenon is that the process of revelation under hypnosis exerts an effect upon the conscious ego. readying it in the interim for the often uncomfortable and unwelcome disclosures which have been made already under trance conditions. This single feature of hypnoanalysis makes the analysis of resistances superfluous, and permits the clinician to come to grips with crucial matters affecting the patient.

Now as the repressed and deflected come to light both in the waking state and in the trance, the therapist can validate the contents of the analysis, can fill in the gaps, and manipulate the analysis so that he is assured of the import and scope of each item. This he can do, if it is necessary, by viewing the material in both situations, and so obtaining a better and well-rounded picture of the problem at hand. He can and must also assure that the entire personality shares in the abreactive process. It is a cardinal principle of hypnoanalysis that abreaction take place in the waking state so that the entire functioning organism will share in the established therapeutic benefit of this process. Under regression and revivification there will appear crucial and dramatic events of biography which are of pathogenic significance. Until the fully integrated organism participates in these, hope of success in therapy is forlorn. As a matter of fact, unless this is accomplished, the essence of hypnoanalysis is lost, and all the negative criticisms which apply to the superficial suggestive therapies will be in order.

Yet another feature of technique for the middle phase must be mentioned. It has been found that often the waking organism is unprepared for the acceptance of material which has been revealed under hypnosis. Because of this, it becomes necessary to follow each episode of trance with post-hypnotic amnesia for the contents of the trance, thus permitting the interim phenomenon to accomplish the ego-preparing work of paving the way for a routine acceptance of such items.

The final phase of therapy is entered upon when it becomes clear that all the factors accounting for the therapeutic problem have been exposed, reacted to, and examined. The transference relationship which has, during the hypnoanalysis to this point, been exploited for continuity of treatment, now becomes the central agent for bringing it to a close. In essence, this final phase is synthesizing and educational. From the exploration of the total organism there will have appeared varied pathology of ideas, goals, and attitudes which have originated in misconceptions, misinterpretations, and from the employment of the various mechanisms of defense. The hypnoanalyst now has as his task to reeducate his patient in respect of all of this, and to exert toward the reorientation of the personality along more hygienic lines. Herein the usual techniques of psychoanalysis are employed, but these are reinforced by post-hypnotic suggestion. More than mere verbal acceptance of the new goals, attitudes, style of life, ways of regarding the past are required by hypnoanalysis. These must literally be incorporated into the performing organism and be shared by it in all the levels and segments of the personality. What is called for is a real engrafting process. At last, the transference relationship is dissolved. This is accomplished by redistributing its energies along the lines indicated by the therapeutic course. Here, again, hypnosis is drawn upon as an agent of enforcement to exert an effect upon those components of the organism not otherwise accessible.

The problem of the operationally effective field for hypnoanalysis has been under examination by me and others during the past few years. At the present writing, it appears that the technique is applicable in every instance where a dynamic investigation of the personality is wanted, and to the treatment of such psychogenic disorders and aberrations in which there is presented to therapy a relatively intact ego.

The categories to which hypnoanalysis has been applied with success are as follows: hysterical somnambulism, anxiety neurosis, homosexuality, alcoholism, kleptomania, schizoid personality, symptomatic asthma, frigidity, adult maladjustment, conversion hysteria, psychopathic personality, problems in adaptation, and pre-psychotic personality types. To this list, workers at the Menninger Clinic add anxiety hysteria, hysterical psychosis, neurotic depression, and psychogenic reaction to pregnancy. The following case history illustrates the application of hypnoanalysis to a patient who suffered from hysterical somnambulism.

HYPNOANALYSIS IN A CASE
OF HYSTERICAL SOMNAMBULISM

The patient was a prisoner in a Federal Penitentiary. He was a young, healthy, serious-minded man who had adjusted very well to institutional routine and who was being considered for a parole. It was decided that since the psychological implications of the case were the major factors involved, the possibilities of treatment should be explored and the question of parole made dependent upon the outcome of such treatment. In spite of the patient's fine institutional record, pleasing personality, serious plans for the future and excellent general attitude, the paroling authorities were reluctant to grant parole if examination disclosed the possibility of future "attacks," or prognosticated further difficulties with the law. The patient himself stated that he preferred to be treated for his condition than to be released under the perpetual shadow of further episodes.

He was accepted by a psychiatric colleague who began a series of treatment interviews. Excellent progress, based upon a gradually developing transference relationship, was made. Unfortunately, the psychiatrist was ordered elsewhere. Before leaving the vicinity, however, he suggested to me that I assume the case, pointing out the patient's suitability for the type of therapy (hypnoanalysis) with which I had been concerned.

The treatment period lasted some three months, M, the patient, appearing daily except Sundays for sessions of one hour. Almost the entire first two weeks were concerned with training in hypnosis. The patient was, in the first two hours, instructed in relaxation on the couch and the fixation of attention on my voice. The remainder of the first week was devoted to achieving a satisfactory depth of the trance state with ease, confidence and rapidity. By the end of this period M was able to reach the desired depth of sleep almost immediately upon my suggestion.

The second week consisted in preliminary attempts at recall. M was first asked to reproduce the events of the instant day, then of the preceding day, then of the preceding weeks. By the close of this second week, the formal history had been recited.

The procedure employed during the three months following the preparatory period cannot be described in detail. Essentially, free-association was the rule for the opening of each hour. When resistances were encountered, M was asked to go to sleep. As soon as it was ascertained that he was in the trance state, his last few associations and recollections before the hypnoidal sleep were given him, and he was asked to continue from there. Then he was given a complete amnesia for what had transpired during that session *after* the associative material of the waking state had ceased flowing. The following day the key associations (that is, those which M had given previous to falling asleep) were again presented.

Hypnosis was employed to disintegrate resistance, to facilitate recall, and also to distinguish between real and screen memories. But perhaps its most dramatic employment was in those sessions where, in order for proper evaluation of early experiences and the recovery of traumatic events of childhood and adolescence, such scenes were recreated *in toto*. Herein it was necessary—and a task of the utmost delicacy—to determine the literal role of the patient. Was he the adult M looking back upon an event and interpreting it in the light of subsequent life-experiences and the distortions of years of attitudinizing, reflecting, and wishing? Or was he the M of the time being portrayed? The test which I have developed from considerable experience with hypnoanalysis to distinguish between what Erickson has so aptly called "regression" and "revivification" is a wholly behaviorial one requiring detailed scrutiny of the way in which the motor apparatus is employed and coordinating the results with known criteria of this apparatus at various developmental stages. (The smoothness with which a pencil is grasped, a shoelace tied, a tie knotted, an object lifted, etc., provides a time-line of almost limitless applicability in such questions.)

Again, hypnosis was used to recover those "lost" periods in M's history; those episodes when, to all intents and purposes, M functioned automatically, amnesiacally. Here also delicacy was called for, as well as continual validation. It was necessary to recapture the flavor of the conditions which obtained immediately previous to such attacks and to attune M to them in such a manner that no discord would wreck the psychological atmosphere so constructed.

Finally, where in the waking state interpretations of behavior in the analytic sense had been arrived at and accepted, the full force of suggestion was brought to bear upon M to insure the actual "grafting" of such altered views and attitudes upon the personality. Through this means was assured the benefits of treatment, and in this way also was the transference finally dissolved, or better, displaced into proper channels.

M, our patient, was born in a small southern town in 1916. Birth was normal, without sequalae to mother or child. Early and subsequent physical development was without special incident. He suffered most of the childhood diseases, from each of which he emerged without apparent damage. Childhood years were, on the surface, happy ones. He entered school at the age of six, completed the elementary course by steady advancement to graduation with an average scholastic and deportment record. In high school his conduct deteriorated and several violations of discipline were noted. This behavior culminated in the destruction of a teacher's classbook in his last high-school year. For this he was expelled, thus bringing his school history to a premature close.

M's parents were fairly typical middle-class southern whites. His mother is a literate, competent, somewhat overburdened housewife who, since the death of her husband, has been dependent upon the children. The father was, by turns, a semi-professional baseball player, a farmer, a repairman for the railroad. He was a rather hearty out-of-doors type, with strong family feeling and considerable pride in his offspring. Until his death in 1935—our patient was almost 19 at the time—he supported his family in an average fashion and had achieved and held a commendable community reputation. Neither the direct nor the collateral family history contains instances of insanity, feeblemindedness, epilepsy, alcoholism or delinquency.

Our patient was the second of five children. He is the only one to have had difficulties with the law. The others all developed normally. His older brother is happily married and holds an excellent position; the next youngest, a girl, is unmarried at 21, an X-ray technician and trained laboratory worker. The two remaining children are still in school.

Home life was apparently congenial. Sexual history began with masturbation at 14. As an adolescent M preferred boys to girls for company. Initial heterosexual experience was at 16, with casual and moderate indulgence up to time of marriage.

In 1935, following expulsion from school and the death of his father, M enlisted in the Marines. He achieved a good service record, sent most of his earnings to his mother, saw service on maneuvers outside the continental limits. He states that he enjoyed the soldierly life, worked hard to become a communications expert.

About a year after enlistment he was brought to the attention of medical officers at his post hospital because of somnambulism. The earliest notation includes the following episode:

"One night M was seen to light his pipe in bed and then smoke for a while. He laid the pipe on the locker and got up and walked out of the building. Several of his bunkmates overtook him and led him back to his bunk. When he awoke they told him what had occurred and he did not remember walking or smoking the pipe."

Because of such nocturnal wanderings M was sent to a Naval Hospital where the following incident, typical of many, was observed.

"Patient had his arm flexed so that his head was resting on the palm of his hand. He was lying on his side with blanket thrown on opposite side of head. He was kicking his feet with a quick motion about once every minute. At 1:35 A.M. patient got up, put on his shoes while sitting on the chair beside the bed. Patient tied his shoelaces very neatly, then put his hands to his temples, kept them there for one or two minutes. At 1:38 patient stood up with his hands and arms outstretched and walked toward the door. When patient got near water fountain he veered toward front door. Patient did not have his arms stretched out after he passed water fountain, until he was about four feet from door. Patient pulled on front door and tried to open it, but after being assisted by Corpsman to leave door he moved away and sat down at the table near the door. Patient then said he wanted to go out and walk around the park. After some further questioning he said he did not have any place to go.

" 'I am not dreaming. I got up of my own accord.'

" 'Is anyone talking about you? Do you have any enemies?'

" 'No.'

" 'Do you know where you are now?'

" 'Yes, I am in the U.S. Naval Hospital.'

" 'What day is it?'

" 'Sunday night.'

"At 1:45 patient got up and tried to open door again. After failing, he walked with a quick step toward door. Turned around, walked to back door of solarium and tried to open it but it was locked. Walked to water fountain, drank some water and with outstretched arms felt his way to bed. Sat down on chair, took off shoes and socks, got into bed and pulled blankets over body, partly covering head.

"At 1:47 patient was awakened by rubbing his face and back of neck with damp towel. Patient awakened, jumped up in bed in a sitting position, swinging arms as if frightened. Patient said, 'What is this? What's the matter?' Then he laughed and said, 'Did I cause any trouble?'

"During all this time, until awakened at 1:47 A.M., patient's eyes were closed tightly. Patient said he did not remember anything after going to bed at 11 P.M."

Following clinical observation of such episodes as that described above, with no known physical disability, M was discharged from the Marine Corps for somnambulism. It was suggested that these episodes may have been precipitated by a desire to leave the Marines for a position in industry which he had been promised.

On leaving the Marines, M worked first at a low-salaried job as a shipping clerk. After a time, however, and as a result of an examination, he secured a position as a railway mail clerk. Six months later he married a local girl. The marriage was unopposed by all save his wife's sister. The couple lived compatibly. His wife soon became pregnant.

At midnight of a summer's day in 1941, M reported for work as usual in the post office. There was only one other clerk on duty that night. At 2 A.M., M received a registered package containing a large sum of money, government bonds, and jewelry, for which he gave a receipt. On turning over the mail to the other man, he was asked about registered mail and specifically stated that there had been none. He left work at 7 A.M. At 1 P.M. the same day he sent a telegram to the authorities reporting the pouch of registered mail as missing.

When the postal inspectors later questioned M he claimed he had no recollection of what had happened. A search of his car, however, revealed more than $1500 in currency. At the local jail, after hearing M's story of sleepwalking, it was suggested he go to sleep and try to remember what had transpired. Some two hours later he fell asleep and apparently while asleep (his eyes were closed) he offered to direct the officers to the stolen articles. He then led them to his mother's farm and showed them the spot where the money was buried. Most of it was recovered in this way. Significantly, however, it was noted that while in this state he was able to dodge holes in the ground and low-hanging limbs of trees.

M was sentenced to a lengthy term in Federal custody. No further episodes were noted (with the exception of those produced under hypnosis) from the time of his admission to his release on parole.

That the hysterical syndrome is built upon a primitive phantasy involving repressed wishes is well-known among analysts and analytic-minded clinicians. The nine formulations of Freud are exhaustive in their review of the psychogenesis of the hysterical reaction; while further contributions have stressed, more or less comprehensively, the expressive nature of the hysterical symptom. Not so well appreciated, however, are the protective aspects of the hysterical manifestation, the dynamics of symptom-formation and, quite as important, the pre-eminence in this variant of deviating behavior of what can best be described as "freedom from guilt."

The case of M provides good if somewhat circuitous illustration of those less understood features of the hysterical syndrome. For M, the flight into somnambulism was a defense against a classical triad. It served (1) as protection against a strong sadistic component, nourished in subliminal memory, and directed initially against his mother, subsequently against all females; (2) as protection against acceptance of forceful homosexual strivings arising from identification with a highly colored father image; (3) as protection against castration anxiety which had its seed in the sado-maso-chistic climax of the phantasy arising from the opposition of the active-sadistic passive-homosexual conflict engendered by (1) and (2).

Perhaps the best approach to our material is the phantasy basic to M's retreat into hysteria. Early in the hypnoanalytic sessions it was possible to obtain a rounded account of it. The scenes, the characters, the words and gestures were always the same from the first phantasy experience at the age of 12 to the time when it underwent the startling change at the age of 17.

It was customary for M to indulge in this phantasy before falling asleep, but it appeared frequently in daydreams as well. He did not rehearse it every night. It would seem that it appeared four or five times during the year. The phantasied scene is a bedroom. A woman, clothed in a colored wrapper, is lying on the bed. A man is standing near a door which opens on a corridor. Across the corridor, M and his older brother are sleeping in a room which resembles exactly the one our patient occupied during childhood. The man and woman are talking loudly, angrily. M awakens, rises from his bed, crosses the hall and enters the room. He enquires of them, "Why are you fighting?" The woman answers, "He's hurting me." M says, "I'll show you what hurting means!" Then he approaches the bed. The woman cowers fearfully. M reaches over and tears off the colored wrapper. Underneath, she is nude. M becomes excited at her nakedness and begins to pummel her with his fists. He is very elated and strikes harder and harder blows, directing them mainly against her buttocks, breasts, and mouth. She cries, "Stop, you're hurting me." The man in the doorway laughs. When M is almost exhausted he turns to the man and says, "Show me what you have." The man obliges by revealing an abnormally long penis. M becomes aroused and sheds his pajamas. Suddenly the man exclaims, "You have no peter! You must be a girl!" and with that the secene ends.

At least, so ended the scene until the radical change at age 17. After that time, it ceased abruptly at the point where the man in the scene revealed his phallus. The feeling-tone in the early version of the phantasy M recalled as one of ecstatic well-being until the final discovery was made, after which there was exhaustion and depression. The later version was always rehearsed in an intensely elated spirit.

The key to the phantasy and subsequently to the chief symptomatic manifestation in the case (as well as to the personality organization of M) was found in the numerous dreams he brought and in the hypnoidal reconstruction of the somnambulistic periods. Some of the dreams which had a direct bearing upon the psychological constellation responsible for the clinical picture follow.

A dream which appeared early in the hypnoanalysis and proved of tremendous importance as an opening wedge in our case was:

"I went into the house and there was only my wife, another woman and a baby. I don't know who the other woman was, but she was holding our baby. The baby seemed to be a little girl, about three years old. I said to my wife, 'I thought you said our baby was a boy.' She answered, 'Well, I thought so too until now.'

"I woke up feeling very tense and nervous."

This dream is a patent admission of underlying homosexuality and of M's concern over it. The woman is, of course, M's mother, M is the (girl-boy) baby. (In point of fact M, at the beginning of the hypnoanalysis, was the father of a boy of 18 months.) The wife's remark is an undisguised reference to M's impotence on the first night of their honeymoon, when, after repeated attempts at penetration, M was too exhausted (so he believed) to consummate the wedding. In his associations to the dream, M seemed to be resentful toward the mother-figure. He questioned her right to hold the child "because she might spoil it," and remarked that if the dream had been longer he might have snatched it from her. He wondered if the woman (Mother) might have been responsible for the transformation of the boy-baby into a girl. As for this child, he expressed considerable relief that it was actually a boy and confessed the prospect of its having been female in the dream caused the tension experienced upon awakening. It was apparent that he identified completely with the baby and that through the medium of the dream he brought into focus one of the fundamental sources of intrapsychic conflict as well as a paramount consideration for later use in solving the phantasy and accounting for the symptom.

Another dream which was even more important since it provided a major clue to the problem was:

"I was in a large room full of men. The room seemed to be as large as our dining hall here. Every man had on a white sleeping gown which reached to his ankles. Everyone was standing up and had a shiny tin plate full of roast beef which he was eating. When a man finished he would fall in line. They all marched past a desk where a woman was accepting contributions for the Red Cross. I was in the crowd, but was only looking at the others. I wanted some roast beef."

Initial association to this dream concerned the prevalence of homosexuality in prisons. The men were all homosexuals, indulging their appetites. The white gowns further symbolized their femininity. *But they had to pay for their indulgence.* Each had to make a contribution to the Red Cross: in short, each had to submit to castration, the only acceptable coin, the only passport to homosexuality. M wished to partake of the roast beef, i.e., engage in homosexual practices, but he was unwilling to pay the price. Finally, it was his mother, the woman at the table, who was to exact the payment. While associating further to the dream elements, M pointed out that the roast beef appeared especially delectable since, as he phrased it, "it seemed to be a special treat because it was not meal time and the men were standing, not sitting as they usually do at meals." He also remarked that contrary to rigid custom in prisons, no custodial officers were on the scene. This he interpreted as license to enjoy the "treat." Furthermore, it was even more unusual for a group of "sex-starved" convicts to be permitted unattended in a room with a woman, and yet "they weren't interested in her at all. No one seemed to have anything to do with her until he had to pay for the meal." The symbolism of the Red Cross was transparently phallic and castrative.

The following dream introduces the father image and hints at the initial identification leading to the repressed homosexual strivings:

"I was in a room with a man who was formerly the chief of detectives in my home town. This man was asked to resign his position for drunkenness, etc. and later he rented trailer space on my mother's property. While we were in the room, he was sitting on a chair and I was standing up. We were arguing. The argument was about my parking my car on the place he had rented for his trailer. Suddenly he made a move which made me think he was going to pull a pistol on me. When he did it a second time, I pulled one on him and shot him. He seemed to slump down in the chair and I got scared. Suddenly, though, he straightened up and laughed at me. I said to him, 'You didn't even try to protect yourself. Didn't you have a gun?' He said, 'Why, certainly, I had one.' He then pulled out two pistols from his pocket. He and I then left this room together and walked up a long, long corridor with our pistols in our hands.

"I awoke in a happy frame of mind and found it had been a wet dream."

The chief-of-detectives is the father who possesses the mother. He at first objects to the boy's intrusion in the parental relationship. M responds by exhibiting his adequacy to take over the father's chief (as M views it) function. The father, however, produces two weapons, thus establishing his dominance. Cementing of a homosexually oriented attachment is symbolized by the march up the long corridor together. Of further interest is M's attempt to deny masculinity to the father and on this basis to question the paternal prerogative. The shooting of the father symbolizes the homosexual intent toward him. Comparisons such as trailor vs. car, two guns vs. one gun, point up the irritating convictions of inadequacy of M.

The fourth dream of special significance in this selection referred to even more remotely repressed anti-female sadism in M. It appeared late in the hypnoanalysis and provided, at last, the missing step in the difficult climb to complete solution of the persistent phantasy.

"I dreamed about Tonto (of the Lone Ranger comic strip). He was trying to track down a gorilla that had been attacking women. Tonto could not track the gorilla because he was going by smell and he had lost the scent. However, he went doggedly until he reached a house. A woman came to the door. She was all beaten up and bruised. She said that the gorilla had come through the window into her bedroom. She said that he had attacked her and beat her up, and that while he was doing this to her she had pulled some of the hair from his body. She had laid these bristles on her pillow. Tonto then rushed into the room to pick up the fresh scent from the hair. They were certainly big thick bristles."

The dream was prophetic. Tonto was the hypnotist, on the trail of information regarding the still deeper motivations of M. The patient was here actually offering what was being sought, and it is most interesting that the surrender of such important material was made in a dream. The woman was again M's mother. The choice of the gorilla to represent himself indicates the baseness with which M consciously regarded the sadistic component as well as the amount of aggressive hostility it comprised. The dream was, of course, a wish fulfillment but it contained as well a castration motif. It repeated the warning knell of other dreams (especially dream #2 of those discussed) that indulgence in and satisfaction of such primitive desires must be paid for by castration, signified by the loss of the hairy bristles.

The material resulting from dream analysis, together with the data from the other phase of the hypnoanalysis, enabled M to interpret the phantasy, account for its genesis historically, and relate it to the symptom formation.

The phantasied woman was the mother originally, womankind later: the phantasied man was the father originally, all males later. The situation was a distortion of confused and confounded memorial elements designed to fulfill strong id wishes generated pro-oedipally. It was founded on the surreptitious observation of the primal scene, suffered grotesque alteration in its reception by an infantile consciousness at a time when the age was in its most pliable and hence plastic stage in the identification process. This led to the introjection of a father image which, while strong, was inadequate to the reality situation from a psycho-sexual point of view; and eventually proved inadequate in superego construction. Hypoanalysis, stressing revivification, recaptured the historic events which, although they were discrete in point of time, nevertheless had jelled to form the phantasy. Visual and auditory participation in the primal scene led to conception of the parental relationship as a debasement of the mother. Since this occurred *before* the primitive son-father struggle for the mother was entered upon, the flow of libido in the direction of the father was never altered, and the homosexual (passive-receptive) identification made continuous. Sadistic orientation of the personality was initiated from the primal scene and a succession of historic episodes which pyramided into a personality inclination exploited by a primitive ego. M was at once the attacker of the mother and passive recipient of the attack. So, there was the identification with the father on a homosexual level, and participation in the sadistically-pleasurable attack (from the infant's place of vantage), and the further identification with the suffering but receptive mother. The latter was inescapable from the developmental point of view since the libidinous organization was in the stage of ambivalence, the libidinous energy streaming bi-directionally. Subsequently, an enforcement of the homosexual and the sadistic elements took place as childhood, pubertal, and early adult years brought novel yet somehow vaguely representative experiences.

The last but equally important member of the triad casts the decisive vote in the formation of the symptom (somnambulism) and completes the phantasy construct. Observation of the "castrated" female in the form of the mother, together with remembrance of submission to the dominant father, plus the castration fancies of infancy and childhood—and further enforced by sibling rivalry with the advent of the next (girl) child—resulted in the conviction that indulging the primitive sin would result in loss of the phallus. Homosexuality, i.e. submission to the father, meant castration. This was the stern, impervious injunction of the demanding super-ego.

Now the phantasy becomes completely intelligible. It runs the dark gamut of the infantile wish and ends with payment for its gratification.

If we now draw upon the revivified hypnoanalytic material relating to the reconstruction of the somnambulistic states and those situations in which the symptom appeared, we understand the genesis and significance of M's behavior. Through hynosis we were able to recover many episodes of hysterical sleepwalking and daytime periods of blankness. A few will serve our purpose here.

At the age of 17 the last part of the phantasy changed radically. The castration theme disappeared. Until that time there had been no sleepwalking, and this fact is supported by a recalled statement of the father to that effect. The first known episode took place on the night of a day when M had been hunting with his father. He reported that they had had a fine companionable outing and had returned in glowing spirits but "all worn out." M went to bed immediately and tried to sleep. He could not. The phantasy returned and acted itself through until the point just previous to the castration motif. M's brother awakened him sometime later. It seems the older boy had returned home from an engagement in town and had come upon M, apparently asleep, wandering aimlessly on the lawn. Revivification recovered the continuity of the phantasy, acting itself out in the sleepwalking state. The companionable outing had signified something more to M. But he could not break through the thought of payment. Hence the falling of the curtain, the "black-out," the "loss of consciousness," at the instant before the wages were inexorably exacted.

M's circumstances in the Marines just before his removal to the Naval Hospital were somewhat similar. He had formed a strong attachment to a fellow serviceman, based apparently upon mutually latent homosexual inclinations. The phantasy appeared almost nightly during this time and, as we know, the episodes of somnambulism were frequent.

One very interesting occurrence during waking hours took place when M was courting his future wife. They had gone to the movies and on their return were sitting on the porch "necking and petting." Suddenly, M arose, walked to his car. The girl, sensing something peculiar in M's behavior, ran after him and clambered into the car just as M started the motor. They drove for about an hour, in complete silence, M staring ahead blankly. Near an airport on the outskirts of a city, M parked the car. For almost an hour he sat staring, while the girl attempted by every means to arouse him. Some time later he "came to," inquiring where they were and what he had been doing. When this episode was revivified it became clear that the ego, fearful of the consequences of sadistic id-impulses generated by the violent stimulation of love-play, and horrified at the prospect of having to pay for such gratification, initiated the retreat into the automatic behavior described.

Unfortunately, we cannot here discuss the episode which contained the commission of the crime leading to M's incarceration. It is enough to indicate that it took place soon after his wife became pregnant; that M was concerned whether the child would be male or female. (Would he "pay" in this way for his latent homosexuality and substitutive possession of the female?) The stolen valuables represented an "insurance" against the "payment" to be exacted; and, finally, the hiding of the money and valuables on the mother's farm carried the usual soiling sadistic connotation.

The function, then, of the hysterical symptom shown by M was protection from the unbearable idea of castration. It was as if the ego literally withdrew and disclaimed all responsibility for the basic id urges, leaving the field to an insistent super-ego which was actually bent on its "pound of flesh." Similarly, the withdrawal of ego from participation served yet another purpose: it freed it from the guilt which attempted to cascade into consciousness as a sequence to such objectionable thoughts as expressed in the precipitating phantasy. Indeed, as in other hysterias, the symptom enabled a modified dissociated state to obtrude itself. The formulation, "Not I (ego) can be held accountable for this. I am not guilty," suits the picture very well. (Further evidence for the guilt-avoiding nature of the hysterical reaction comes from the study of multiple personalities especially under hypnosis. A patient exhibiting hysterical paralysis of an arm put it most succinctly recently when he said to me, "It's not me: it's my arm!")

The case of M, an hysterical somnambulist, serves as a vehicle for discussing the technique of hypnoanalysis. The basic phantasy in this case was a triad of latent homosexuality, sadism, and castration-anxiety; composed pre-oedipally, and transformed into symptom. The somnambulistic symptom has been shown to function as a protective mechanism employed by the ego to escape the consequences of deeply entrenched id-urges and super-ego punitive demands. A further function of the symptom was the avoidance of and freedom from guilt. The method of hypnoanalysis, apart from its usefulness as a time-saver which radically shortens the treatment period, was especially helpful in achieving abreaction, since it entailed literal revivification. The results achieved were brought about by a carefully interwoven combination of hypnosis and free-association periods which brought to the surface repressed materials, validated beyond doubt the substrata of awareness, and embedded firmly as accretions to the personality, the analytic interpretations and significances arrived at by the patient's own efforts.

WILL HYPNOTISM

REVOLUTIONIZE MEDICINE?

BY

DR. S. J. VAN PELT

Lest the reader should form the wrong conclusion from the title of this article, let the writer hasten to explain that he would be the very first to deny that hypnotism is a panacea for all human ills. Nevertheless, it is hoped to show that there is a far greater scope for its use in medicine than is generally recognized.

Nobody, no matter how fanatically he may be opposed to hypnotism, can deny that in this science we have the most powerful and effective method of controlling the mind and, through the mind, the whole body. When a few words by suggesting paralysis, for instance, can render a hypnotized person powerless to move, although fully conscious and able to reason, who can doubt the power of hypnotism? When hypnotic suggestion can cause the mouth to water, change the heart rate or cause the sweat glands to function, who can fail to be impressed with its possibilities in medicine?

More and more is heard these days of the influence of the mind in medicine and recently, in an article in the British Medical Journal entitled "In Praise of Idleness,"[1] the importance of the role it plays in the so-called "stress diseases"—thyrotoxicosis, duodenal ulcer and non-renal hypertension—was pointed out. Again, in another article "The Mind and the Skin,"[2] in a different issue of the same Journal, a long list of skin diseases was given in which the psychogenic factor was stated to play a part. This list included such conditions as acarophobia, dermatitis factitia, trichotillomania, neurodermatitis, pruritus ani and vulvae, atopic eczema, rosacea urticaria, hyperidrosis, cheiropompholyx, seborrhoeic dermatitis, psoriasis and alopecia areata!

Nevertheless, in these articles, although the importance of the mental factor was clearly shown, no mention was made of the most effective method of controlling the mind. Treatments advocated and discussed varied from major operations to divorce, and giving up work, but the simplest of all treatments, that of medical hypnosis, was not even considered. What is the reason for this attitude? Mainly, of course, it is due to the fact that hypnotism has been given a bad name as the result of crude but spectacular stage performances. One can hardly blame a doctor for hesitating to recommend hypnotism to a patient, for the latter would, more often than not, recoil in horror at the suggestion. Stage performances, often in very bad taste, blatant and wildly extravagant claims of medically ignorant amateur hypnotists, sensational stories of the Svengali-Trilby type, lurid articles in the Press, foolish radio plays with "master criminal hypnotists," and the "occult" flavor imparted by those who imagine themselves to be "psychic," have all combined to present hypnosis as something to be feared and shunned as "not quite nice" by the majority of people, lay or professional.

Almost as bad is the credulous belief of those who are impressed by the antics of a few stage "stooges" and who fondly imagine that it is only necessary for the hypnotist to exert his "amazing power" to "force" the patient to give up his symptoms. Such people regard hypnotism as some sort of "magic" and consider that it is sufficient to say "hocus pocus, now you're well," in order to cure anything from ingrowing toenails to decayed teeth.

Before it can be hoped to make progress with the use of hypnosis in medicine, these foolish ideas must be corrected and hypnosis stripped of all its nonsensical and mysterious trappings, so that it can be presented as a simple, serious and straightforward method of medical treatment. As a first step towards this, some indication of how it "works" must be given. At lectures to B.M.A. Divisions, for instance, the writer has often been asked "How is it that one method of treatment can help cases so widely different?" Doctors are naturally, and quite rightly, suspicious of anything which claims to be a "universal cure." The field in which hypnosis can be useful is so wide that, at first sight, it may appear like claiming that some new "wonder drug" will cure everything.

However, when the matter is examined more closely, it will be seen that there are sound scientific reasons for using hypnosis in such widely varying conditions. Nobody would deny the importance of the automatic nervous system and the part it plays in regulating the functions of the body. No organ or gland can work without the appropriate orders from this system. Similarly, nobody can deny that in hypnosis there is a greatly increased control over the autonomic nervous system. This is not just a matter of theory, for such control has been scientifically demonstrated. Even in the waking state it is possible to influence the autonomic system by suggestion. It is well known that it is possible to bring "tears to the eyes" or "make the mouth water." Suitable suggestions can make a person blush or feel angry, sad, happy or afraid and often evoke all the bodily symptoms which accompany these conditions. Of all the phenomena which can be evoked in hypnosis, the one which is common to all stages, even the lightest, is *increased suggestibility*. Thus we can see that, in hypnosis, even the lightest, we have an *increased control over the autonomic nervous system* and, indirectly, of all the organs and glands it supplies.

This complex system supplies all those muscles and glands which are not under voluntary control and normally it achieves the desired results without any conscious effort on our part at all.

Such vital processes as the heart action, activity of the sweat glands or digestive processes and dilatation or contraction of the bronchi and blood vessels are all under its influence. This whole system, with everything it controls, is *profoundly influenced by emotion,* so that it is easy to see how vital functions of the body can be affected by hypnotic suggestion. As Fulton[3] says, "The heart and circulation may be worked just as hard and just as much as a detriment to the body as a whole from an armchair . . . as from a rower's seat."

With a proper understanding of the above, it becomes more

understandable how such widely varying conditions as those described in the following cases can benefit from hypnosis. One factor is common to all of them and that is FEAR—and fear, no matter of what it may be, produces a disturbance of the autonomic nervous system. Resultant physical symptoms frighten the patient still more until a vicious circle is established. The patient literally becomes "afraid of the symptoms of fear." Hypnosis, properly used, can break this vicious circle and, by enabling the patient to really listen to calming and reassuring suggestion, restores the balance of the autonomic system with a consequent disappearance of unpleasant symptoms. Consider the following typical cases:

1. *Restoration of hair color and growth.* The patient, a young married woman, suffered a severe accident. Shock and worry caused the hair to turn white and fall out "in handfuls." The patient developed *a great fear* of baldness and the loss of her husband's affection. After several sessions of hypnosis, she was able to adopt a calmer and more philosophical attitude. Some months later she was able to report restoration of normal growth and color of her hair. Such a result may appear incomprehensible until it is remembered that fright, through its action on the autonomic, can cause blood to be withdrawn from the skin—in this case the scalp —with consequent lack of nourishment to the hair.

2. *Migraine.* This young man reported with a history of severe attacks of migraine over a period of eight years. The condition began while studying for an important examination in which he feared failure. *Fear of the condition,* which had resisted all orthodox methods, including injections, had kept it going. Several sessions of hypnosis with reassurance and relaxation were sufficient to bring about a cure.

3. *Insomnia.* The patient, a middle-aged man, reported that he had been unable to sleep without heavy doses of drugs for years. The condition followed a period of worry and anxiety over business and domestic affairs. *Fear that insomnia would lead to "madness"* had kept it going. Several sessions of hypnosis during which he was reassured and shown how to relax properly, were sufficient to enable him to sleep without drugs.

4. *Anxiety state.* A middle-aged married man complained of severe trembling, sweating and palpitations and a feeling "as

though his inside was turning over" at the slightest excitement. The condition followed a shock at the sudden death of a relative, when the patient developed a great *fear of death* himself. Explanations and reassurance during several sessions of hypnosis were sufficient to enable him to regain his normal confidence.

5. *Asthma.* This patient, a young man, reported that he had suffered from asthma every night for years.

Following a heavy, indigestible meal, he had awakened one night and felt "unable to get his breath." *Fear of this unpleasant feeling* had done the rest. After several sessions of hypnosis, he was able to relax completely and sleep naturally, with consequent disappearance of his asthma.

6. *Blushing.* The patient, a businessman, reported that he had blushed ever since he had been made a fool of by a superior during his early days at work. *Fear of looking foolish* had so disturbed the balance of his nervous system that he blushed at the slightest provocation. A few sessions of hypnosis were sufficient to enable him to control his feelings easily, with consequent disappearance of the habit.

7. *Sexual frigidity.* The patient, a young married woman, reported that her fear of sex, resulting from unfortunate experiences as a child, prevented her living a normal married life. Explanation and reassurance under hypnosis enabled her to develop normal feelings towards her husband and after a few treatments she reported that everything was satisfactory. Such a case is easily understandable when it is remembered that *fear,* acting through the autonomic system, inhibits sexual feeling.

8. *Sexual impotence.* The patient, a middle-aged man, reported with this complaint, which had followed a period of worry and anxiety. *Intense fear* of the condition had kept it going. A few sessions of hypnosis, during which the true nature of the condition was explained, were sufficient to restore the patient's confidence with consequent disappearance of the complaint.

9. *Enuresis.* The patient, a young man, reported that he had wet the bed every night since childhood. He was bitterly ashamed of the condition and was literally *afraid to go to sleep.* After a few sessions, during which it was explained that fear had kept the condition going, his confidence was restored and he reported some time later that he now slept perfectly dry.

10. *Intermenstrual hæmorrhage.* The patient, a young married woman, reported that she had suffered excessive bleeding between the periods for several years. The condition, which had followed a domestic upset, had resisted all medical treatment and although nothing organic could be discovered, the operation of hysterectomy had been advised. After a few treatments *she lost her fear* of the condition and the periods became normal. An accident some time later caused some irregularity but this was corrected with a few more sessions of hypnosis. It is common knowledge that suggestion can influence the menstrual cycle. Why not use it scientifically in appropriate cases?

Even in cases of bad habits such as alcoholism or excessive smoking, hypnosis can help. Such conditions are usually a result of an attempt on the part of the patient *to ease nervous tension* and seek relief from its unpleasant effects on the autonomic nervous system. Consider the following typical cases:

11. *Alcoholism.* The patient, a married man. complained that he had got into the habit of taking excessive alcohol because he felt *"all strung up"* owing to excess of work. *Fear of alcoholism* only made him worse. When the patient was shown how to relax properly and reassured under hypnosis, he reported himself free of the habit after a few sessions.

12. *Excessive smoking.* The patient, an elderly man, suffered from severe bronchitis and had been advised to give up his heavy smoking. He was unable to do this and *feared the ill effects on his health.* A few sessions of hypnosis by removing his fear and enabling him to relax were sufficient to free him from the habit.

When it is remembered that conditions such as these, and a host of others which are closely allied to them, all respond very simply to hypnotic suggestion, it becomes obvious that there is a very real place in medicine for this valuable method of treatment.

Once prejudice has been overcome and the tremendous scope of hypnotism is realized, then we may expect to see a veritable "revolution" in medicine. Then, no doubt, patients with insomnia will no longer be merely "doped" with sleeping tablets, but referred to a properly qualified hypnotist for the appropriate treatment.

Those who doubt that "mere words" can ever take the place of drugs should consider the facts put forward in an article "Drug Action and Suggestion" in a recent issue of the British Medical Journal.[4] Here it was stated that "clinically the action of the drug can be profoundly modified by numerous factors arising from the vagaries of the intact patient" and further that "the human body reacts not only to physical and chemical stimulation but also to the symbolic stimuli of words and events which have acquired a special significance for the individual."

HYPNOTHERAPY
FOR VOICE AND SPEECH DISORDERS

JOHN J. LEVBARG, M.D.

As a rule disorders of the voice and speech mechanism are functional in character and psychic in origin. It is up to the physician
to seek the proper causes producing such a disturbance before he
can look for a cure.

My work in this field has been conducted at the Harlem Eye
and Ear Hospital and in my private practice. The most common
disorders encountered were stammering and stuttering. The terms
stammering and stuttering are used interchangeably by some speech
pathologists, but to distinguish them from the layman's point of
view, stammering is a condition in which one cannot start, whereas
stuttering is a repetition of sound—in other words, one gets started
but cannot stop. With either disorder the patient is neurotically
inclined, anxious and fearful, and the speech mechanism is momentarily paralyzed. This paralysis may be due to a spasm of either
the throat, lips, glottis or respiratory muscles. The patient cannot
think clearly while speaking to another, is always on the watch
for words he thinks he cannot say, speaks rapidly, feels embarrassed
and self-conscious and cannot adjust himself adequately. In a great
majority this effect is accompanied by complete somatic contrac-

tions, tensions, spasms, twitchings, clenching of the jaw or blinking of the eyes. In my opinion the defect is not in making the beginning sounds but in relaxing the muscles for one moment in time to produce the next. Rarely is there blocking or repetition of a consonant at the end of a syllable. Other speech and voice defects in this group were dysphonia pubetica, i.e., a high-pitched falsetto voice, and hysterical aphonia, in which there was either a total loss of the voice or a condition producing merely breaks in the rhythm. Spastic and choreic speech were also considered for experimentation. Choreic speech is largely due to a motor disability with a great deal of uncoordinated movement of the speech organs.

One of the greatest drawbacks for complete success with all these patients is the consciousness of introversion. Such persons admit an inadequacy and manifest a negative condition which is vital to progress and success. I have found that suggestion in the waking state is not readily accepted, but when it is remembered that hypnosis is the art of mentally controlling the thoughts and actions of a patient, one can realize the great value it possesses to those who employ it in the practice of correcting speech disorders.

Hypersuggestion can be readily used, as most of these persons suffer from various forms of nervousness which have no actual cause for their existence. Their morbid self-consciousness severely interferes with their success in life. They are especially excessively nervous in the presence of strangers. Some have cold perspiration over the entire body, the heart beats rapidly, the voice falters, respiration fails them, and they are a picture of confusion. Hypnosis is greatly instrumental in strengthening the morale of these victims and in helping them to meet the exigencies of everyday life. It is absolutely necessary to ingrain in the mind the feeling of adequacy and equality, and all sense of inferiority in the presence of strangers and acquaintances must be removed.

The importance of instilling a new habit in the mind of such a person is essential. Every one knows that every move or voluntary action is controlled by one's thoughts, and this continued nervous force makes definite imprints on the brain tissue. When this nervous energy is repeated, lasting impressions are made, and thereafter the action practically becomes almost involuntary. This agrees with Pavlov's experiments on conditioned reflexes in dogs. By repeatedly emphasizing a certain action in the same manner, a lasting impression is established in the dog.

Under hypnosis a patient with a speech disorder readily becomes passive and receptive, and his psychic resistance is easily overcome. When the speech pathologist suggests thoughts of recovery, thus making positive ideas penetrate the mind, the patient readily believes symptoms no longer exist or that they will disappear. One is instilling faith and confidence in the patient and is reenforcing constructively the physical, mental, moral, social and economic status of such a person. In other words, the brain accepts and transforms suggestions into a reality. This belief becomes fixed and is not easily diverted by negative waking suggestions.

The following cases, selected from the group of various forms of speech disorders, demonstrate the response to the practical application of hypnosis.

REPORT OF CASES

CASE 1.   Samuel S., a youth aged 18, came to the clinic from April 17th until October 9th. His condition was diagnosed as dysphemia clonica, a substitution of sound and oral inactivity. He went through elementary school in ungraded classes. While his mental level as determined by the Stanford-Binet test was low, this was not believed to be an entirely valid measure of his true mental ability. His shyness, poor speech and poor language background have all probably contributed to make his score low. At an examination with tests involving mechanical ability he did much better, being only somewhat below average. His speech defect was a serious handicap to eventual vocational placement. At the second session he was directed to lie on the couch and to gaze fixedly at a chrome-plated pencil having a round globe tip. He was told to think of sleep and not to resist the physician. In less than three minutes he entered the cataleptic stage, and then posthypnotic suggestions were given. He was seen once a week, and within a month marked improvement in speech was noted. Before he stopped coming to the clinic he obtained a position as a clerk in a grocery store and was getting along splendidly.

CASE 2.   W. W., a shipping clerk aged 24, a stammerer, was first seen early in August at my office. He complained of fear of speaking before strangers. The fear caused a severe dull headache, which was constant and unbearable. Under hypnosis the headache was relieved immediately. The patient received three treatments per week, and within a month correction in speech was evident. At the time of writing the patient is enthusiastic, can speak before strangers and is also able to read before a group. He was going to study for the ministry, but he felt his speech defect to be a serious handicap. He now has renewed ambition to carry out his original intention, and he expects to take up his studies this summer.

CASE 3.   Miss S. F., aged 41, a music teacher, came to my office late in September. Owing to emotional shock, her voice would break, and she was unable to sustain a phrase but for a few seconds. Her speech would block, crack and become jerky, sometimes it was entirely disturbed. The patient is hypertense and easily upset. Weekly sessions under hypnosis inspired confidence and better control of the voice.

CASE 4.   H. M., aged 16, came to the voice and speech clinic on January 16th, with a high-pitched falsetto voice. He was nervous, shy and diffident. Physical examination gave negative results. He had had a deviated septum corrected for sinus trouble. Under waking suggestion the voice dropped one octave at the first session, and at the third session the voice was fuller, vibrant and a man's voice. Under hypnosis nervousness improved. In this case visits to the clinic were irregular, and in late October he was discharged as cured.

AUTOHYPNOSIS
AND HABIT CONTROL

BY

ANDREW SALTER

The great value of hypnotism in habit formation is one of the main reasons for the psychological interest in hypnosis. Hypnotism, of course, can be used in the treatment of various phobias, shyness, nailbiting, stuttering, and many other selected conditions.

Some years ago I published methods whereby it is possible to hypnotize oneself. The interested reader can find them reported in detail.[1]

At this point I should like to explain briefly the techniques of autohypnosis before I consider their application to habit formation. The first method is essentially autohypnosis by posthypnotic suggestion. In this technique the hypnotist determines if the person who wishes to learn autohypnosis is a good hypnotic subject. If limb catalepsies or glove anesthesias can be produced, it will be found that it is possible to teach the subject autohypnosis. A limb catalepsy of some sort, or an inability on the part of the subject to get out of the chair, is prerequisite to the successful application of this method.

The qualified subject is then told that in a few minutes he will be hypnotized and while in a trance will be given posthypnotic suggestions dealing with hypnosis: "I will tell you that whenever you wish to hypnotize yourself, you have merely to sit or lie down as comfortably as you can, and let the thought flash through your mind that you wish to hypnotize yourself. You will take five deep breaths, and on the fifth breath you will be in the deepest possible trance, and then you will give yourself whatever suggestions you wish, and wake up whenever you want to. Every time you wake from a trance you will feel fine—splendid." The essence of the rest of the technique is essentially this: to explain to the subject that it does not matter who gives him the suggestions—suggestions will be effective as long as the subject wants them to be effective. The source of the suggestions is unimportant. They may come from within or without. "As long as you cooperate with me, or with yourself, the suggestions will work. And that is the way it will be when you hypnotize yourself."

The other two methods of autohypnosis are essentially as follows: A good hypnotic subject is given typed autohypnotic material which parallels the hypnotic suggestions that were previously found effective with him. There is no point in giving a complete verbatim example, for the directions vary from case to case. The illustrative material that follows is composed of a few typical cross-sections of what the subject is instructed to memorize at home, at leisure, and while wide-awake. It reads, in part, something like this:

I feel very comfortable. My arms are so relaxed. My feet feel very relaxed and heavy. I feel so very comfortable and relaxed. My whole body feels comfortable and relaxed. I just want to sleep. I feel so comfortable.

My eyes are getting heavy, so very heavy. They're closing bit by bit, they feel so heavy and relaxed. I feel them closing more and more. I want to sleep, and I want my eyes to close.

It will be noted that the instructions to be memorized are tantamount to the usual hypnotic instructions. Toward the end, the instructions read:

Now I am fast asleep, in the deepest possible hypnotic sleep. I am in a deep sleep, as deep as the deepest hypnotic sleep I have ever been in. I have complete autohypnotic control of myself. I can give myself autohypnotic suggestions, and awaken whenever I wish. I can talk to the person who gave me these autohypnotic instructions, yet I will still remain fast asleep. I will follow such instructions as he gives me, yet I shall still have autohypnotic control.

The subject is told to memorize these instructions, and not to concentrate too much on their meaning. He is told that he may paraphrase them if he wishes. The subject is also told, however, not to try to hypnotize himself with these instructions until the hypnotist has gone over the instructions with him and shown him how to apply them.

The last method of autohypnosis might be called "fractional autohypnosis." Here again we need a person in whom it has been possible to produce, by waking suggestion, a limb catalepsy or an inability to get out of the chair. The subject is then taught to autosuggest lightness, heaviness, warmth, and cold to his hands and to his feet. Each sensory modality is worked with separately. Then hypnotist and subject, working together, mix autohypnosis with heterohypnosis, and the subject is taught to bring himself into a deep trance. *In this trance the subject can give himself suggestions and awaken at will.*

Here then, in their essence, are three techniques for producing autohypnosis. It is indeed an interesting question to ask ourselves why these methods are effective.

Every word has associations. Just as Pavlov's dogs learned to salivate at the sound of a bell—because that bell had been associated with meat—so do good hypnotic subjects respond to the words uttered to them by the hypnotist. Words are the bells of conditioned reflexes. Through persistent associativities from infancy, the word "cloud" means "cloud," and in fact has a "cloud-like quality." As Watson said,

"We must dislodge the age-old belief that there is some peculiar essence in words as such. A word is just an explosive clutter of sound made by expelling the breath over the tongue, teeth, and lips whenever we get around objects. We condition our children to make the same explosive sounds when they get around the same objects."

Words are the bells of associative reflexes. Such words as "splendid," "marvelous," and "magnificent" give us an unconscious lift because we have been conditioned to that feeling in them. The words "hot," "boiling," and "steam" have a warm quality because of their associativity. Inflection and gesture have been conditioned as intensifiers of word conditionings.

We can thus see that words are bound up with completely unconscious associative reflexes. Certain words in an appropriately trained person can produce actual bodily sensations, or more broadly, actual bodily reactions.

How convenient it would be to say that the phenomena of hypnosis are "caused" by "suggestion," but such a meaningless explanation has beset hypnotism for years. How much simpler and more meaningful it is to realize that hypnosis is based on associative reflexes that use words as the triggers of automatic reactions. Hypnosis is the production of reactions in the human organism through the use of verbal or other associative reflexes.

Hypnosis basically involves conditioned reactions and reflexes. Some people have conditionings which we can evoke to create the so-called "trance" state. In this state it is possible to give verbal conditionings to be carried out on the occurrence of an after-awakening "bell"—so-called posthypnotic suggestion.

Since hypnosis is based on *verbal habits,* the use of hypnosis in habit formation is a logical consequence of the most elementary nature. I think this point is worth mentioning, for many of the critics of the use of hypnosis and autohypnosis in habit formation are apparently unaware of the close relation of hypnotic theory to habit formation. With hypnosis we substitute good habits for poor ones, for logically considered, personality is nothing but a broad system of habits.

Keeping in mind the fact that personality is a broad hierarchy of habits, let us see the application of autohypnosis to a case of migraine.

Here is a young woman, age 29, who complains of migraine headaches. She has been to see a procession of physicians, and all have assured her that it is "all in her mind." She has the intent, listening quality, and the superficially relaxed appearance that is usually found in excellent hypnotic subjects (those who have had experience with hypnosis will know precisely what I mean), and I decide to dispense with any preliminary tests of suggestibility, by which I mean dispensing with the use of Chevreul's pendulum and the falling-back test.

After a minute and a half of direct hypnotic suggestion her eyes close, and her head falls to the side with a jerk. I stop the suggestions and have her open her eyes. She expresses the usual surprise and amazement at all this, and I then go into detail, explaining to her what I plan to do: to wit, that I will hypnotize her and develop her into an excellent hypnotic subject, after which her hypnotizability will be used to teach her autohypnosis. (The reader will note that we are using Method I, that is, autohypnosis by the use of posthypnotic suggestion.)

I then go through the standard hypnotic procedure with her, and she responds quite well, to the extent of having a full amnesia on awakening, and also, at my suggestion, a posthypnotic visual hallucination of Gilbert Stuart's portrait of George Washington on a blank page of a book I show her.

In further sessions with me she was taught, by posthypnotic suggestion, to take five deep breaths, on the fifth of which she would be in a deep trance. She was also taught, through posthypnotic suggestion, to produce headaches in herself at will, and also to be able to shut them off at will. She was further taught to give herself suggestion about a generally more relaxed attitude toward people and situations, and a generalized freedom from worry. And that is all there was to her migraine.

I would like to make some comments about this case. Note, for example, that she was an excellent subject for hypnosis. This made teaching her autohypnosis an absolute certainty. Note also that instead of giving her a generalized autohypnotic self-control, some *limited specific objectives* were taught to her. Neglect of this point is often responsible for the failure of autohypnosis to achieve the most dramatic results. This is an extremely important point. It is best to mold specific objectives into the subject. This may also be done more obliquely by having the subject, in the standard post-hypnotic way, do several of the things that the subject will afterwards be called upon to do autohypnotically. If the subject has had certain *hetero*hypnotic experiences, even though they are not auto-hypnotic to him, it will be found that the subject will be able to apply these specific suggestions by himself.

The subject should be warned against using autohypnosis to produce positive or negative visual or auditory hallucinations, for the successful achievement of this can be most confusing to a subject. It is possible to give posthypnotic suggestion blocking the capacity of the individual to do this, but it is not necessary. In general, the heterohypnotic stage is used to mold the particular form that the autohypnotic control will take.

In general, the key to the understanding of autohypnosis is an understanding of heterohypnosis, and an awareness of the fact that all that autohypnosis involves is a shift in the point of origin of the suggestions. All of the principles and cautions of hypnosis remain the same. But the fact that the hypnotic results are pro-duced by the subject himself, permits the subject to overcome the diminishing effects of the usual posthypnotic suggestions. The sub-ject overcomes this diminished power of posthypnotic suggestion by giving himself autohypnotic suggestions as often as necessary. As a result, these autohypnotic suggestions become ingrained in his mind and become habitual. And when these suggestions have become sufficiently ingrained, autohypnotic suggestion is no longer necessary. The individual has acquired habit control through auto-hypnosis.

SELF-TAUGHT AUTOHYPNOSIS
FOR INSOMNIA AND OBESITY

RAPHAEL H. RHODES

———————————

Warren's "Dictionary of Psychology" defines hypnosis as: "An artificially induced state, usually (though not always) resembling sleep, but psychologically distinct from it, which is characterized by heightened suggestibility, as the result of which certain sensory, motor, and memory abnormalities may be induced more readily than in the normal state." C. L. Hull, in his "Hypnosis and Suggestibility," contends that hypnosis is a state of relatively heightened susceptibility to prestige suggestion. Andrew Salter, in "What Is Hypnosis," says that hypnosis is "an aspect of conditioning." In "Hypnosis: Theory, Practice, and Application," I wrote: "Hypnosis may be defined as a condition in which a shift in the relative positions of the subjective and objective minds has been consummated, and in which the subjective has been brought to the fore with the expectation of being controlled either by the hypnotist or by the recessive objective. The process which achieves this result is hypnotism. When it is induced by a hypnotist, and the subjective advances with the expectation of being controlled by the hypnotist, it is called hypnotism by external control. When the subject himself induces the subjective-objective shift, and the subjective advances with the expectation of being controlled by the recessive objective, the process is called autohypnotism or autohypnosis."

All authorities agree that hypnosis involves some type of mental adjustment in the subject. Usually this mental adjustment is directed by another person, called the hypnotist, and the subject enters the trance state with the expectation of being controlled by that hypnotist. Autohypnosis, developed by Andrew Salter, involves a variant form of mental adjustment in which the direction toward trance is autonomous, and the subject enters the trance state with the expectation of remaining in control himself. Salter's "Three Techniques of Autohypnosis," which first appeared in the 1941 *Journal of General Psychology,* describes how a subject may be taught to hypnotize himself and give himself suggestions with post-hypnotic effect.

The technique of autohypnosis can be learned by the average person. Once he has mastered autohypnosis, he can modify his habits and attitudes, and regulate his appetites and desires through this device. In the control of insomnia, which is more often due to faulty psychological patterns than to disturbed physiological processes, autohypnosis has been effective. Obesity due to compulsive overeating has also been treated successfully by the same means.

Previously published techniques of autohypnosis rely upon the presence of a hypnotist during the learning process, either to give posthypnotic suggestions or to direct and integrate various phases of the method. Any new skill, whether it be swimming, tennis, chess, or autohypnosis, is more easily learned under the guidance of a competent teacher. Each of these skills, however, may be mastered through reading and practice alone, without the actual presence of an instructor.

Consider swimming, for example. The instructor supplies much more than a description of how to breathe, kick, and stroke. He also supervises the manner and extent of the practice sessions, remains on hand to correct mistakes, and gives encouragement when the pupil's courage falters. Nevertheless, one may learn to swim without the presence of an instructor, if he will follow printed directions meticulously, practice diligently, and work with the conviction that correct and thorough application of the printed directions will bring success. The absence of an instructor, however, does impose a special burden of application and practice upon the student.

So, also, it is possible for a serious student to master autohypnosis without the presence of a teacher-hypnotist. A person who is eager to teach himself autohypnosis can do so by reading and following carefully the instructions given below.

The first stage of autohypnosis is "eye closure." By this I mean a condition in which, although you are awake, you cannot open your eyes. It may be achieved as follows: Sit in a comfortable chair, in a quiet room. Then:

1. Say *one* and as you say it, think, "My eyelids are getting very, very heavy." Repeat that thought, think only that thought, concentrate upon it, mean it and believe it as you think it. Exclude any other thoughts such as, "I'll see if this will work." Just repeat the one thought, "My lids are getting very, very heavy." If you think only that thought, concentrate upon it, mean it and believe it as you think it, your lids will begin to feel heavy. Don't wait until they get very heavy. When they begin to get heavy, proceed to the next step.

2. Say *two* and as you say it, think, "My eyelids are getting so heavy now, they'll close by themselves." As in *one,* repeat that thought, think only that thought, concentrate upon it, mean it, believe it. Do not force your eyes closed, do not fight to keep them open; just concentrate on the one thought, "My eyelids are getting so heavy now, they'll close by themselves," and as you repeat that thought, that thought alone, let your eyelids do as they want to. If you really concentrate on that thought to the exclusion of any other, mean it and believe it as you think it, your eyelids will slowly close. When your lids are closed, allow them to remain shut and continue as follows:

3. Say *three* and as you say it, think, "My lids are so tightly shut, I cannot open them no matter how hard I try." As above, repeat that thought, think only that thought, concentrate upon it, mean it and believe it. As you do so, try to open your eyes and you will find that you cannot until you say the word *open,* and then your lids will pop open.

Do not be discouraged by failure in your first attempts at self-taught autohypnosis. This is the type of experiment in which the average person will fail the first two or three times he tries it. That is because the average person has not learned how to concentrate upon one thought alone, that is, to the exclusion of all others. This is not due to a lack of intelligence. Indeed, intelligent people have rather involved thought patterns and are accustomed to thinking more than one thought at a time. Concentration upon only one thought, to the exclusion of all others, involves a new discipline, and this requires determination and practice. So, if you fail the first time, try again. If you are intelligent enough to control your mental processes, you can succeed in thinking only one thought at a time; and once you achieve that ability, autohypnosis is in your grasp.

Thus when your eyes close after *two,* and you go on to *three* and think, "My lids are so tightly shut, I cannot open them no matter how hard I try," you must keep repeating that thought, that thought alone, and as you think it, try to open your eyes.

As long as you concentrate on that thought alone, your eyelids will remain shut. Your muscles will strain to open them, but your eyes will remain shut until you say *open,* either out loud or mentally.

Once you have achieved eye closure, the next step is to speed up the process. Try it two or three times to make sure the eye closure is good. Every time you do it, the effect will be stronger. Now for the acceleration. Do *one* as above, and the moment your lids get heavy, go on to *two.* As you say *two,* think the requisite thought only once, or twice at most, but think it exclusively. By now you will have acquired that ability. As your lids close, say *three,* and again think the requisite thought only once, or twice at most, but think it exclusively. Your lids will remain shut. Release them by the command, *open.*

Now go through the procedure once again, but instead of saying *one, two,* and *three,* just think those numbers, following each one with its appropriate thought. Finally go through the entire procedure without the numbers; just think the thought for *one* once, the thought for *two* once, and then the thought for *three* once. With practice you may be able to get almost instantaneous eye closure by merely letting your lids close and thinking the thought for *three* once.

You will find that as you acquire speed, you achieve stronger and stronger control. Having mastered the discipline of concen-

trating upon one simple thought at a time (steps *one* and *two*),
you will be able to attain step *three*, a complex thought, almost
instantaneously. The touchstone of your success with autohypnosis
is rapid eye closure. Once you have achieved that, you can proceed
to the depth of trance necessary to meet your particular problem
or problems.

The next step is relaxation. Keep your eyes closed, and think,
"I'm going to take a deep breath and relax all over." Take a
deep breath, and as you exhale you will relax all over. Think,
"I'll breathe normally and deeply and relax more and more with
every breath." After that, as you breathe, you will relax more and
more.

With good eye closure and relaxation (which in a short time
comes with the eye closure), you will have attained the first degree
of autohypnotic trance. Your mind is now ready to accept suggestions you make to it with both hypnotic and posthypnotic effect. But
just as in the case of the eye closure itself, where the total rapid
result was built up through repetition. so also the succeeding steps
sometimes need practice. The secret of success is concentration—
the ability to think one thought at a time, to the exclusion of all
others, and to mean and believe it.

Try simple suggestions first. For example: Grasp your left index
finger with your right fist. Think, "I cannot pull my finger out."
As above, concentrate on that thought alone, mean it, believe it,
and as you think it, try to pull your finger out. It will remain stuck
until you think, "Now I can release it," or use some other word or
phrase with similar import. Extend your right hand in front of
you; make a fist. Think, "My arm is rigid like a steel bar; I cannot
bend it no matter how hard I try." As you think that, try to bend
it and it will remain stiff until you think *relax* or some other similar command. Interlock your fingers, palms together, and think,
"My fingers are stiff and rigid. My hands are stuck together; I cannot pull them apart no matter how hard I try." As you think it,
try to pull them apart, but they will remain stuck together until
you release them by a specific appropriate command. You can then
try, "My feet are rigid; I'm stuck to the chair; I cannot stand up."
While you think it, try to stand up and you will not be able to do
so until you utter or think a specific appropriate command.

You can also control sensory reactions. Concentrate on your right hand. Think, "It's getting numb from the wrist down. All sensation of pain has gone from it. It has no feeling, just as if it were covered by an asbestos glove instead of skin. It's absolutely painless." As you think that, pinch it with your left hand, and you will find that your right hand is numb, insensitive to pain. If it continues to register pain, that is because you did not concentrate sufficiently. (Remember, the eye closure did not work the first time either, but now you have it.) Try it again. Concentrate on the thought of insensitivity to pain, on that thought alone, mean it, believe it. If you do, you will achieve glove anaesthesia. You can test the degree of anaesthesia by pinching your left hand with your right, and observing the difference. Once you achieve glove anaesthesia, you can control the sensation of pain in any part of your body by the same method.

Never use this ability to mask any organic difficulty. Pain is a danger signal, a warning. Treating the pain without treating the underlying cause of it will mean serious trouble. Consult your physician or dentist about any organic condition with symptoms of pain.

You can control other sensations also. Think, "My right hand is getting warm, very, very warm." Concentrate on that thought and your right hand will get warm while the left remains unaffected. Try it with your feet. You can make one foot warm and the other cold at the same time.

Some people respond better to suggestions involving sensation (warmth, pain, etc.) than they do to those pertaining to muscular reactions (arm rigidity, finger grasp, etc.). You may respond to both equally well, or perhaps poorly to both. Do not be discouraged if the response is poor. It may be due to your failure to concentrate sufficiently; practice and application will improve your ability. Success in one phase enhances the confidence which is requisite for success in the other phases also.

In any event, once you have achieved good eye closure rapidly, you can proceed to overcome insomnia or obesity even without first obtaining the sensory or motor responses described above.

INSOMNIA

The chief characteristic of insomnia is the insistent recurrence of one or more thoughts besetting the mind. Insomnia is generally the result of a pattern established over a long period of time. If you can achieve good eye closure rapidly, you can use the same power of concentration to force sleep to come to you. Proceed as follows: Lie in bed in any comfortable position. Get eye closure. Then think, "I'll take a deep breath and relax all over." Relax on the exhalation. Now think, "I'll sleep soundly and wake up well." Breathe deeply. Inhale as you think, "I'll sleep soundly." Hold your breath for a moderate time. As you exhale, relax, and think, ". . . and wake up well." Repeat that pattern of breathing and concomitant thought process; only that, nothing else; mean it, believe it. If you do, it will work every time.

Another method of combating insomnia is the following. It may be used either in a chair or in bed, but preferably in bed. Close your eyes, and think, "My feet are getting heavy, very heavy." When they begin to feel heavy, "Now my arms are beginning to feel heavy, very heavy." When the arms begin to feel heavy, "Now my whole body is getting heavy, very, very heavy. I'm going to go deep, deep, deep to sleep." After a slight pause, "My feet are heavy now, very, very heavy." When they feel heavy, "My arms are heavy now, very, very heavy." As you become conscious of the reaction in them, "My whole body is heavy now, very, very heavy. I'm going deep, deep, deep to sleep." After a slight pause, "I'm so relaxed, my eyes are tightly closed. I cannot open them even if I try." With your eyes closed, roll your eyeballs up as if you were looking through your forehead. Try to open your lids. They will remain shut. Take a deep breath and relax on the exhalation. Think, "My feet are getting numb and rigid. I cannot move them." Concentrate on that thought, that thought alone, mean it, believe it, as above explained. If you do so, you will not be able to move your feet. Then immobilize your arms in the same way. Now you are ready to put yourself to sleep. Think, "I'll sleep soundly and wake up well." Adjust the two phrases of that sentence to inhalation and exhalation as above explained. Repeat the pattern of breath and thought to the exclusion of anything else, and sleep will shortly follow.

Although not part of the technique of autohypnosis, there are a few additional suggestions which may be helpful to the insomniac. 1) Breathe deeply. Deep breathing is conducive to relaxation; relaxation leads to sleep. Moreover, the concentration on the process of breathing deeply helps dispel other thoughts. 2) Make notes. Keep a pad and pencil at your bedside. If a recurrent thought disturbs you, perhaps because you want to remember it in the morning, make a note of it. Once the notation is made, your mind will more readily become calm. 3) Be comfortable. Attend to your wants: get a warm blanket if you need it; adjust the window as you wish; eat a cracker if you are hungry; drink if you are thirsty. Don't lie and think about these things. Do them, and forget them. Leave your mind clear to concentrate on one sentence only, "I'll sleep soundly and wake up well."

OBESITY

Obesity (i.e. excess weight) is more often caused by overeating than by glandular imbalance. Obesity cannot be controlled by autohypnosis, but overeating can be. The appetite can be controlled. If it is, the weight will diminish. The less you eat, the less you will weigh. But if your intake remains the same, no amount of autohypnosis will charm away your excess fat.

Appetite, like other habits, grows by what it feeds on. The increase in the habit of overeating, however, goes beyond the simple laws of use. Overeating is sometimes a compensating device for the satisfaction of psychological hungers as well as physical ones, and as such it may be compulsive in nature. Furthermore engorgement itself results in the enlargement of the stomach, which in consequence naturally demands more food the next time. Thus overeating is a vicious circle. On the other hand, a diminution of intake results in gradual shrinking of the stomach with consequent lessening of appetite.

To combat obesity, you must destroy the old habit of overeating, and establish a new habit of moderation instead. Through autohypnosis you can do this successfully because you will be working in a positive rather than in the usual negative way. Autohypnosis enables you to suggest to yourself that foods of high caloric value are distasteful, and it also enables you to autosuggest a feeling of satiety even when you have eaten little.

Once you have secured good eye closure through either of the methods described above, you may proceed to give yourself suggestions. Think, "I don't like starchy or fatty foods, butter, chocolate, cream, and heavy desserts. They make me bloated and uncomfortable." Repeat that thought. If you concentrate upon it while in the trance state, it will have a posthypnotic effect upon your appetite. You may add, "I will enjoy lean meats, fruits and vegetables. They taste good, and will make me feel strong and well." In point of fact, present-day researches are implicating fatty, very rich foods as possible causative factors in arteriosclerosis and heart disease, which take such a high toll of our well-fed population annually. It is not necessary to say all this to yourself every time you try autosuggestion for appetite control. Once you realize it, however, the phrases outlined above will have added potency for you.

At first you will, nevertheless, feel hungry. That is because your abnormally enlarged stomach demands more than an average amount of food. To overcome the sensation of hunger until your stomach contracts to normal size again, use autohypnosis to control its reactions. Follow the securing of eye closure with autosuggestions of warmth to the right hand, to the left hand, to either foot. Make these limbs cold, or warm, upon command. Then autosuggest that your stomach feels cool, empty, and hungry. When you can produce that sensation at will, think, "When I say *that's enough,* my stomach will feel warm, satisfied, and full." If you have learned how to concentrate as above described, you will be able to produce the desired sensations in any limb or part of your body upon command. Condition your stomach to react to the words *that's enough* by feeling warm, satisfied, and full. Once the reaction is automatic, you can produce it also at the table. When you know you have eaten enough, but still feel hungry, say *that's enough;* your stomach will react as it has been conditioned to, and the meal will be over.

As explained earlier in this article, the absence of a teacher imposes a special responsibility upon the pupil. In the absence of a critic and guide to correct and encourage, you must perform those functions yourself. You must be teacher as well as learner. Determination and application will prove rewarding.

Once you have mastered the techniques of autohypnosis, you may use them not only for the control of insomnia and obesity, but for many types of self-improvement. The discipline of concentration, which is an inherent part of the learning process, remains a valuable asset. The ability to make various kinds of suggestions with posthypnotic effect is a powerful psychological instrument for good. Through it, you can achieve relaxation and equanimity, increase concentration, improve memory, and develop self-control. With intelligent use of autohypnosis, you can improve your personality and strengthen your character at will.

NOTES AND REFERENCES

HYPNOSIS: WHAT IT IS AND WHAT IT DOES

1 Cf. the Theory of Psychic Relative Exclusion in HYP-
   NOSIS: THEORY, PRACTICE AND APPLICATION
   by Raphael H. Rhodes (Citadel Press, New York, N.Y.).

2 *Time* magazine, September 2, 1946 issue under Medicine.

HYPNOSIS IN RECONDITIONING

Originally appeared as part of a chapter, Hypnosis in
Psychobiologic Therapy, in Vol. II of MEDICAL HYP-
NOSIS, published by Grune & Stratton, Inc., which kindly
granted permission for use of the material in this volume.

1. JONES, M. C.: The Case of Peter, *Ped. Sem.* 31: 308-318,
   1924.

2 YATES, D. H.: An Association Set Method in Psychotherapy, *Psychol. Bull.* 36: 506, 1939.

3 MAX, L. M.: Conditioned Reaction Technique; a Case
   Study, *Psychol. Bull.* 32: 734, 1935:

4 MOWRER, O. H., and MOWRER, W. M.: Enuresis—
   A method for its Study and Treatment, *Am. J. Orthopsychiat.* 8: 436-457, 1938.

5 LEUBA, C.: The Use of Hypnosis for Controlling Varia-
   bles in Psychological Experiments, *J. Abnor. & Soc.
   Psychol.* 36: 271-274, 1941.

6 PLATANOW, K. I.: The Word as a Physiological and
   Therapeutic Factor, *Psikhoterapiya* 11: 122, 1930.

HYPNOSIS AND ALCOHOLISM

Originally appeared in *The British Journal of Medical
Hypnotism,* which kindly granted permission for use of the
material in this volume.

HYPNOTIC CONTROL OF MENSTRUAL PAIN

Modified from the article entitled The Psychosomatic Treatment of Functional Dysmenorrhea which originally appeared in the *American Journal of Obstetrics and Gynecology*, Vol. 46, No. 6, Dec. 1943, which kindly granted permission for use of the material in this volume.

HYPNOTHERAPY FOR CHILDREN

Modified from the article entitled Psychological Treatment in a Child Guidance Clinic, which originally appeared in the Autumn 1951 edition of the *British Journal of Medical Hypnotism,* which kindly granted permission for use of the material in this volume.

HYPNOSIS IN OBSTETRICS

Modified from the article entitled An Objective Evaluation of Hypnosis in Obstetrics which originally appeared in the *American Journal of Obstetrics and Gynecology,* Vol. 59, No. 5, May, 1950, published by C. V. Mosby Co., which kindly granted permission for use of the material in this volume. The authors wish to express their thanks to Mrs. Marie Hopkins, Superintendent of Maternity Hospital, Minneapolis, for her cooperation in this study.

1   GOODDRICH, F. W., and THOMAS, H.: *Am. J. Obst. & Gynec.* 56: 875, 1948.

2   SCHULTZE-RHONHOF, F., *Zentralbl. f. Gynak.* 46: 247, 1922.

3   KROGER, W. S., and DeLEE, S. T.: *Am. J. Obst. & Gynec.* 46: 655, 1943.

4   KROGER, W. S., and FREED, S. C.: *Am. J. Obst. & Gynec.* 46: 817, 1943.

5   GREENHILL, J. P.: YEAR BOOK OF OBSTETRICS AND GYNECOLOGY, Chicago, 1944, The Year Book Publishers, Inc., p. 169.

6   KROGER, W. S.: *Am. J. Obst. & Gynec.* 52: 409, 1946.

7   WOLBERG, L. R.: MEDICAL HYPNOSIS, New York, 1948, Grune & Stratton, Vol. I, pp. 411-413.

8   LeCRON, L. M., and BORDEAUX, J.: HYPNOTISM TODAY, New York, 1947, Grune and Stratton, pp. 248-251.

HYPNOSIS AND SUGGESTION IN OBSTETRICS

Originally appeared in the *British Medical Journal,* May 21, 1949, which kindly granted permission for use of the material in this volume.

HYPNOSIS IN GYNECOLOGIC DISORDERS

Modified from the article entitled The Treatment of Psychogynecic Disorders by Hypnoanalysis which originally appeared in the *American Journal of Obstetrics and Gynecology,* Vol. 52, No. 3, Sept., 1946, which kindly granted permission for use of the material in this volume.

HYPNOTIC TREATMENT OF A CASE OF ACUTE HYSTERICAL DEPRESSION

Originally appeared as The Successful Treatment of a Case of Acute Hysterical Depression by a Return under Hypnosis to a Critical Phase of Childhood in the *Psychoanalytic Quarterly* (Vol. X, No. 4, Oct. 1941), which kindly granted permission for use of the material in this volume.

1 These two points are of special interest to analysts who are accustomed to demand of their patients an awareness of their illnesses and of the need for treatment, and an acceptance of the therapeutic relationship to the analyst. While this is a valid basis for therapeutic work with many of the neuroses it is an impossible goal in dealing with many neurotic characters and with those neuroses which are accompanied by severe affective disturbances, and with psychoses. The analyst who becomes too completely habituated to his own method may delude himself with the idea that his passivity is pacifying, and may overlook the extent to which it may be an assault in terms of the patient's unconscious emotional reactions. The approach described above, therefore, is an illustration of a method whereby, under appropriate circumstances, these difficulties can be circumvented.

2 Here again is an interesting and significant departure from analytic technique in which the implicit and sometimes explicit challenge is to break through every repression. The rigidity with which this axiom of analytic

technique is applied may account for some analytic failures, and also may be an example of conflict between research and therapeutic purposes.

3   MILTON H. ERICKSON: A Study of Clinical and Experimental Findings on Hypnotic Deafness; (1) Clinical Experimentation and Findings, *J. of General Psychology,* XIX, 1938, pp. 127-150.

4   MILTON H. ERICKSON: The Induction of Color Blindness by a Technique of Hypnotic Suggestion, *J. of General Psychology,* XX, 1939, pp. 61-89.

5   The search backwards towards reliving an earlier period in the life of a hypnotic subject occurs in either of two ways. First there can be a "regression" in terms of what the subject as an adult believes, understands, remembers or imagines about that earlier period of his life. In this form of "regression" the subject's behavior will be a half-conscious dramatization of his present understanding of that previous time, and he will behave as he believes would be suitable for him as a child of the suggested age level. The other type of "regression" is far different in character and significance. It requires an actual revivification of the patterns of behavior of the suggested earlier period of life in terms only of what actually belonged there. It is not a "regression" through the use of current memories, recollections or reconstructions of a bygone day. The present itself and all subsequent life and experience are as though they were blotted out. Consequently in this second type of regression, the hypnotist and the hypnotic situation, as well as many other things, become anachronisms and nonexistent. In addition to the difficulties inherent in keeping hypnotic control over a total situation, this "deletion" of the hypnotist creates an additional difficulty. It is not easy for the hypnotist to enter into conversation with someone who will not meet him until ten years hence. This difficulty is overcome by transforming the hypnotist into someone known to the patient during the earlier period, by suggesting that he is "someone whom you know and like, and trust and talk to."

Usually a teacher, an uncle, a neighbor, some definite or indefinite figure belonging to the desired age period is selected automatically by the subject's unconscious. Such a transformation of the hypnotist makes it possible to maintain contact with the subject in the face of the anachronism mentioned above. Unfortunately many investigators of "hypnotic regression" have accepted as valid that type of "regression" which is based upon current conceptions of the past; and they have not gone on to the type of true regression in which the hypnotic situation itself ceases and the subject is plunged directly into the chronological past.

6 The phrase, "It would make mother sick," may have had much to do with her illness: Mother had had intercourse and died. Her friend, who was a mother substitute, had intercourse and died. The same thing was about to happen to the patient. Mother has said it and it must be true. It is a child's passive acceptance of logic from the image with which it has become identified.

7 Here is an important bit of profound unconscious psychological wisdom. The commands had been repeated incessantly in the patient's mind, whether or not in reality they had been repeated as incessantly by the mother. This repetition which is the essence of all neurosis (8) must occur because of the resurgent instinctual demands. Hence the patient indicates in the word "always," her continuing secret insurrection against a continuing prohibition, and therefore her ever-present state of fear.

8 LAWRENCE S. KUBIE: A Critical Analysis of the Concept of a Repetition Compulsion, *Int. J. Psa.*, XX, 1939, pp. 390-402.

HYPNOTIC PSYCHOTHERAPY

Originally appeared in *The Medical Clinics of North America*, May, 1948, New York Number, published by W. B. Saunders Company, which kindly granted permission for use of the material in this volume.

INDUCED HYPNAGOGIC REVERIES FOR THE RECOVERY
     OF REPRESSED DATA
Originally appeared as The Use of Induced Hypnagogic
Reveries in the Recovery of Repressed Amnesic Data in the
Bulletin of the Menninger Clinic (Vol. 7, Nos. 5 and 6, Sept.
—Nov. 1943), which kindly granted permission for use of
the material in this volume.

1 FARBER, L. H., and FISHER, C.: An Experimental
   Approach to Dream Psychology through the Use of
   Hypnosis, *Psychoanalytic Quar.*, 12: 202-216, 1943.

2 ERICKSON, M. H., and KUBIE, L. S.: The Translation
   of Cryptic Automatic Writing of One Hypnotic Subject
   in a Trance-like Dissociated State, *Psychoanalytic Quar.*,
   9: 51-63, 1940.

3 SILBERER, H.: Bericht uber Eine Method, Gewisse
   Symbolische Halluzinationsercheinungen Hervorzurufen
   und Beobachten, *Jahrbuch fur psychoanal. Forschungen.*
   Bd. I., 513-525, abstracted by L. Blumgart, *Psychoanalytic
   Review*, 3: 112. Symbolik des Erwachens und Schwellen-
   symbolik Uberhaupt, *Jahrbuch fur psychoanal. Forschungen*, Bd. III, 621-660, abstracted by L. Blumgart, *Psychoanalytic Review*, 8: 431-433, 1921.

4 SIDIS, BORIS: An Experimental Study of Sleep, *Jour.
   Abnorm. Psychol.*, 1908, 3: 1-32, 63-96, 170-207; and AN
   EXPERIMENTAL STUDY OF SLEEP, Boston, R.
   Badger, 1909, p. 106.

5 KUBIE, L. S., and MARGOLIN, S. G.: A Physiological
   Method for the Induction of States of Partial Sleep, and
   Securing Free Association and Early Memories in Such
   States, *Trans. Am. Neurol. Assoc.*, 1942.

6 KUBIE, L. S., and MARGOLIN, S. G.: An Apparatus for
   the Use of Breath Sounds as a Hypnagogic Stimulus, *Am.
   Jour. Psychiat.*, 1943.

7 JACOBSON, EDMUND: PROGRESSIVE RELAXA-
   TION, Chicago, Univ. of Chicago Press, Second Edition, Revised, 1942.

8 KUBIE, L. S., and MARGOLIN, S. G.: The Process of
   Hypnotism and the Nature of the Hypnotic State, *Am.
   Jour. Pschiat.*, 1943.

HYPNOTIC RELAXATION AND ANALYSIS

Modified from the articles entitled Hypno-Synthesis which originally appeared in the *Journal of Nervous and Mental Disease,* Vol. 109, No. 1, Jan., 1949, and Brief Psychotherapy of the Sex Offender which originally appeared in the *Journal of Clinical Psychopathology,* Vol. 10, No. 4, Oct., 1949, both of which kindly granted permission for use of the material in this volume.

1 The sentence in brackets was added by the editor.

HYPNOANALYSIS

Modified from an article on Hypnoanalysis by Dr. Lindner in the *Encyclopedia of Psychology* published by Citadel Press, and Hypnoanalysis in a Case of Hysterical Somnambulism which originally appeared in the *Psychoanalytic Review,* Vol. 32, No. 3, July, 1945, both of which kindly granted permission for use of the material in this volume.

WILL HYPNOTISM REVOLUTIONIZE MEDICINE?

Originally appeared in *The British Journal of Medical Hypnotism,* which kindly granted permission for use of the material in this volume.

1 OGILVIE, SIR HENEAGE: In Praise of Idleness, *British Medical Journal,* April 16, 1949.

2 SNEDDON, I. B.: The Mind and the Skin, *British Medical Journal,* March 19, 1949.

3 FULTON, J. F.: Cerebral Regulation of Autonomic Function. Proc., *Inter-State Postgrad. Med. Assemb. N.A.,* 1936A.

4 *British Medical Journal,* October 7, 1950, Drug Action and Suggestion.

HYPNOTHERAPY FOR VOICE AND SPEECH DISORDERS

Modified from Hypnotherapy which originally appeared in *The New York Physician,* and Hypnosis: A Potent Therapy For Certain Disorders of Voice and Speech which originally appeared in the *Archives of Otolaryngology,* the publishers of each of which respectively kindly granted permission for use of the material in this volume.

CONTRIBUTORS

MILTON ABRAMSON, M.D., PH.D., Obstetrician and Gynecologist, Minneapolis, Minn. Chief of the Dept. of Obstetrics and Gynecology, Mt. Sinai Hospital, Minneapolis, Minn.; Instructor, Dept. of Obstetrics and Gynecology, University of Minnesota; Attending Physician, Department of Obstetrics and Gynecology, Minneapolis General Hospital; Lecturer in Obstetrics, Hamline University School of Nursing. Author of Anesthetic Aspiration, Asphyxia as a Cause of Maternal Mortality and Morbidity, *Journal Lancet*, Jan. 1945; Breast Feeding the Newborn: Evaluation of a New Technic of Breast Care, *General Practice Clinics*, Oct. 1947, 318-330; Diagnostic Problems Following Abortion, *Journal Lancet*, June 1950; and Hypnosis in Obstetrics and Its Relation to Personality, *Personality*, Vol. 1, No. 4 Nov. 1950.

GORDON AMBROSE, L.M.S.S.A., Child Psychiatrist, London, Eng. Assistant Psychiatrist and Senior Registrar, Prince of Wales Hospital, Tottenham, London, Eng.; Late Medical Officer and Psychiatrical Registrar, Banstead Hospital, Sutton, Surrey; and Hon. Psychiatrist, Park House Approved School, Nr. Guildford Eng. Author of The Value of Hypnotic Suggestion in the Anxiety Reactions of Children, *British J. of Med. Hypnotism*, 2, 20, March, 1951; Hypnotherapy in the Treatment of the Delinquent Child, *Ibid.*, 3, 56, March, 1952; The Technique and Value of Hypnosis in Child Psychiatry, *Ibid.*, 1, 19, March, 1950; and Techniques of Abreaction, *British Medical Journal*, 2 496, August, 1951.

JACOB H. CONN, M.D., Psychiatrist, Baltimore, Md. Assistant Professor of Psychiatry, Johns Hopkins University School of Medicine; Psychiatrist, Johns Hopkins Hospital; Adjunct Attending Neuropsychiatrist, Sinai Hospital; Consultant in Psychiatry, U.S. Public Health Service and in the United States District Court. Author of Psychotherapy in General Practice, *Bull. of the School of*

Med., Univ. of Maryland, 18: 98, 1934; Sexual Curiosity of Children, *Am. J. Dis. Child,* 60: 1110-1119, Nov., 1940; The Treatment of Fearful Children, *Am. J. Orthopsychiat.,* 11: 744-751, Oct., 1941; Psychogenic Factors in Diseases of Digestion, *Gastroent.* 9: 399, Oct., 1947; Psychogenesis and Psychotherapy of Insomnia, *Jr. Clin. Psychopath.* 11: 85, April, 1950; etc.

MILTON H. ERICKSON, M.D., Psychiatrist, Phoenix, Arizona. Chief Psychiatrist, Research Service, Worcester State Hospital, Worcester, Mass. (1930-34); Director of Psychiatric Research and Training, Wayne County Gen. Hospital, Eloise, Mich. (1934-48); Assoc. Professor of Psychiatry, Wayne University College of Medicine; Visiting Professor, Clinical Psychology, Michigan State College. Author of 37 articles on hypnosis, including: Concerning the Nature and Character of Post-Hypnotic Behavior (with E. M. Erickson), *Journal of Gen. Psychol.,* Jan. 1941, Vol. 24, No. 1; The Successful Treatment of a Case of Acute Hysterical Depression by a Return under Hypnosis to a Critical Phase of Childhood (with L. S. Kubie), *The Psychoanalytic Quarterly,* Oct. 1941, Vol. X, No. 4; Hypnotic Investigation of Psychosomatic Phenomena: Psychosomatic Interrelationships Studied by Experimental Hypnosis, *Psychosomatic Medicine,* Jan. 1943, Vol. X, No. 1; The Method Employed to Formulate a Complex Story for the Induction of an Experimental Neurosis in a Hypnotic Subject, *Journal of Gen. Psychol.,* 1944, Vol. 31; etc.

S. CHARLES FREED, M.D., Endocrinologist, San Francisco, Calif. Adjunct in Medicine, Mount Zion Hospital, San Francisco, Calif. Formerly Instructor at the Loyola University School of Medicine. Co-author of PSYCHOSOMATIC GYNECOLOGY (W. B. Saunders, Philadelphia, Pa.).

WILLIAM T. HERON, PH.D., Certified Psychologist, Minneapolis, Minn. Professor of Psychology, University of Minnesota. Author of CLINICAL APPLICATIONS OF SUGGESTION AND HYPNOSIS (Chas. C. Thomas, Springfield, Ill.).

WILLIAM S. KROGER, M.D., Obstetrician and Gynecologist, Chicago, Ill. Assistant Clinical Professor of Obstetrics and Gynecology,

Chicago Medical School. Co-author of PSYCHOSOMATIC GYNE-COLOGY (W. B. Saunders, Philadelphia, Pa.).

LAWRENCE S. KUBIE, M.D. Psychiatrist, New York, N.Y. Clinical Professor of Psychiatry, Yale University School of Medicine, New Haven, Conn.; Faculty, New York Psychoanalytic Institute, New York, N.Y. Author of PRACTICAL AND THEORETICAL ASPECTS OF PSYCHOANALYSIS (International Universities Press, New York, N.Y.).

JOHN J. LEVBARG, M.D., Psychiatrist, New York, N.Y. Assistant Attending Neuropsychiatrist, City Hospital, New York, N.Y.; Medical Director of the Voice and Speech Department, Harlem Hospital E. E.; Attending Neuropsychiatrist, Clinic Welfare Island Disp.; Consultant LaLo-Phoniatrist, Israel Orphan Asylum. Author of Psychogenic Factors in Otolaryngolical Diseases; Failures in Psychiatric Treatment; Learn to Relax with Hypnosis; Hypnosis: A Useful Therapy to Physicians and Dentist; etc.

ROBERT M. LINDNER, PH.D., Psychoanalyst, Baltimore, Maryland. Chief Consultant Criminal Psychologist to the Maryland State Board of Correction. Author of REBEL WITHOUT A CAUSE (Grune & Stratton, New York, N.Y.), STONE WALLS AND MEN (The Odyssey Press, New York, N.Y.) and PRESCRIPTION FOR REBELLION (Rinehart and Company, U.S.A., and Victor Gollancz, England).

GEORGE NEWBOLD, M.R.C.S., D.R.C.O.G., M.M.S.A., Obstetrician and Gynecologist, London, Eng. House Surgeon, St. George's Hospital, Hyde Park Corner, London, S.W.1; Medical Registrar, Bethnal Green Hospital, London, E.2; Resident Obstetrician and Gynecologist at St. Mary's Hospital, Portsmouth, and Paddington Hospital, London, W.9, Orsett Lodge Hospital, Essex. Author of Medical Hypnotism in Modern Therapeutics, *Nursing Mirror;* The Use of Hypnosis in Obstetrics, *British Journal of Medical Hypnotism;* The Importance of Hypnotism in Midwifery, *Ibid.;* Hypno-relaxation Classes in Ante-natal Clinics, *Ibid.;* and Toxaemia of Pregnancy with Central Placenta Praevia, *British Medical Journal;* etc.

RAPHAEL H. RHODES, Psychologist. New York, N.Y. Member of the New York Academy of Sciences. Author of HYPNOSIS: THEORY, PRACTICE AND APPLICATION (Citadel Press, New York, N.Y.).

ANDREW SALTER, Psychologist, New York, N.Y. Member of the New York Academy of Sciences. Author of CONDITIONED RE- FLEX THERAPY (Farrar, Straus & Young, New York, N.Y.); THE CASE AGAINST PSYCHOANALYSIS (Henry Holt, New York, N.Y.); and WHAT IS HYPNOSIS (Richard R. Smith, New York, N.Y.).

S. J. VAN PELT, M.B.B.S., Psychiatrist, London, Eng. President of the British Society of Medical Hypnotists and Editor of the *British Journal of Medical Hypnotism.* Author of HYPNOTISM AND THE POWER WITHIN (Skeffington & Son, London, Eng.).

LEWIS R. WOLBERG, M.D., Psychiatrist, New York, N.Y. Assist- ant Clinical Professor of Psychiatry, New York Medical College, New York, N.Y. Author of HYPNOANALYSIS and of MEDICAL HYPNOSIS (Grune & Stratton, New York, N.Y.).

INDEX

A PERSONAL WORD FROM MELVIN POWERS
PUBLISHER, WILSHIRE BOOK COMPANY

Dear Friend:

My goal is to publish interesting, informative, and in-spirational books. You can help me accomplish this by answering the following questions, either by phone or by mail. Or, if convenient for you, I would welcome the opportunity to visit with you in my office and hear your comments in person.

Did you enjoy reading this book? Why?

Would you enjoy reading another similar book?

What idea in the book impressed you the most?

If applicable to your situation, have you incorporated this idea in your daily life?

Is there a chapter that could serve as a theme for an entire book? Please explain.

If you have an idea for a book, I would welcome discussing it with you. If you already have one in progress, write or call me concerning possible publication. I can be reached at (213) 875-1711 or (818) 983-1105.

Sincerely yours,

MELVIN POWERS

12015 Sherman Road
North Hollywood, California 91605

MELVIN POWERS SELF-IMPROVEMENT LIBRARY

ASTROLOGY
____ ASTROLOGY: HOW TO CHART YOUR HOROSCOPE *Max Heindel*   3.00
____ ASTROLOGY AND SEXUAL ANALYSIS *Morris C. Goodman*   5.00
____ ASTROLOGY MADE EASY *Astarte*   3.00
____ ASTROLOGY MADE PRACTICAL *Alexandra Kayhle*   3.00
____ ASTROLOGY, ROMANCE, YOU AND THE STARS *Anthony Norvell*   4.00
____ MY WORLD OF ASTROLOGY *Sydney Omarr*   7.00
____ THOUGHT DIAL *Sydney Omarr*   4.00
____ WHAT THE STARS REVEAL ABOUT THE MEN IN YOUR LIFE *Thelma White*   3.00

BRIDGE
____ BRIDGE BIDDING MADE EASY *Edwin B. Kantar*   10.00
____ BRIDGE CONVENTIONS *Edwin B. Kantar*   7.00
____ BRIDGE HUMOR *Edwin B. Kantar*   5.00
____ COMPETITIVE BIDDING IN MODERN BRIDGE *Edgar Kaplan*   4.00
____ DEFENSIVE BRIDGE PLAY COMPLETE *Edwin B. Kantar*   15.00
____ GAMESMAN BRIDGE—Play Better with Kantar *Edwin B. Kantar*   5.00
____ HOW TO IMPROVE YOUR BRIDGE *Alfred Sheinwold*   5.00
____ IMPROVING YOUR BIDDING SKILLS *Edwin B. Kantar*   4.00
____ INTRODUCTION TO DECLARER'S PLAY *Edwin B. Kantar*   5.00
____ INTRODUCTION TO DEFENDER'S PLAY *Edwin B. Kantar*   3.00
____ KANTAR FOR THE DEFENSE *Edwin B. Kantar*   5.00
____ KANTAR FOR THE DEFENSE VOLUME 2 *Edwin B. Kantar*   7.00
____ SHORT CUT TO WINNING BRIDGE *Alfred Sheinwold*   3.00
____ TEST YOUR BRIDGE PLAY *Edwin B. Kantar*   5.00
____ VOLUME 2—TEST YOUR BRIDGE PLAY *Edwin B. Kantar*   5.00
____ WINNING DECLARER PLAY *Dorothy Hayden Truscott*   5.00

BUSINESS, STUDY & REFERENCE
____ CONVERSATION MADE EASY *Elliot Russell*   4.00
____ EXAM SECRET *Dennis B. Jackson*   3.00
____ FIX-IT BOOK *Arthur Symons*   2.00
____ HOW TO DEVELOP A BETTER SPEAKING VOICE *M. Hellier*   3.00
____ HOW TO MAKE A FORTUNE IN REAL ESTATE *Albert Winnikoff*   4.00
____ HOW TO SELF-PUBLISH YOUR BOOK & MAKE IT A BEST SELLER *Melvin Powers* 10.00
____ INCREASE YOUR LEARNING POWER *Geoffrey A. Dudley*   3.00
____ PRACTICAL GUIDE TO BETTER CONCENTRATION *Melvin Powers*   3.00
____ PRACTICAL GUIDE TO PUBLIC SPEAKING *Maurice Forley*   5.00
____ 7 DAYS TO FASTER READING *William S. Schaill*   3.00
____ SONGWRITERS' RHYMING DICTIONARY *Jane Shaw Whitfield*   6.00
____ SPELLING MADE EASY *Lester D. Basch & Dr. Milton Finkelstein*   3.00
____ STUDENT'S GUIDE TO BETTER GRADES *J. A. Rickard*   3.00
____ TEST YOURSELF—Find Your Hidden Talent *Jack Shafer*   3.00
____ YOUR WILL & WHAT TO DO ABOUT IT *Attorney Samuel G. Kling*   4.00

CALLIGRAPHY
____ ADVANCED CALLIGRAPHY *Katherine Jeffares*   7.00
____ CALLIGRAPHER'S REFERENCE BOOK *Anne Leptich & Jacque Evans*   7.00
____ CALLIGRAPHY—The Art of Beautiful Writing *Katherine Jeffares*   7.00
____ CALLIGRAPHY FOR FUN & PROFIT *Anne Leptich & Jacque Evans*   7.00
____ CALLIGRAPHY MADE EASY *Tina Serafini*   7.00

CHESS & CHECKERS
____ BEGINNER'S GUIDE TO WINNING CHESS *Fred Reinfeld*   5.00
____ CHESS IN TEN EASY LESSONS *Larry Evans*   5.00
____ CHESS MADE EASY *Milton L. Hanauer*   3.00
____ CHESS PROBLEMS FOR BEGINNERS *edited by Fred Reinfeld*   2.00
____ CHESS SECRETS REVEALED *Fred Reinfeld*   2.00
____ CHESS TACTICS FOR BEGINNERS *edited by Fred Reinfeld*   4.00
____ CHESS THEORY & PRACTICE *Morry & Mitchell*   2.00
____ HOW TO WIN AT CHECKERS *Fred Reinfeld*   3.00
____ 1001 BRILLIANT WAYS TO CHECKMATE *Fred Reinfeld*   4.00
____ 1001 WINNING CHESS SACRIFICES & COMBINATIONS *Fred Reinfeld*   4.00
____ SOVIET CHESS *Edited by R. G. Wade*   3.00

COOKERY & HERBS

_____ CULPEPER'S HERBAL REMEDIES *Dr. Nicholas Culpeper*	3.00
_____ FAST GOURMET COOKBOOK *Poppy Cannon*	2.50
_____ GINSENG The Myth & The Truth *Joseph P. Hou*	0.00
_____ HEALING POWER OF HERBS *May Bethel*	4.00
_____ HEALING POWER OF NATURAL FOODS *May Bethel*	3.00
_____ HERB HANDBOOK *Dawn MacLeod*	3.00
_____ HERBS FOR COOKING AND HEALING *Dr. Donald Law*	2.00
_____ HERBS FOR HEALTH—How to Grow & Use Them *Louise Evans Doole*	4.00
_____ HOME GARDEN COOKBOOK—Delicious Natural Food Recipes *Ken Kraft*	3.00
_____ MEDICAL HERBALIST *edited by Dr. J. R. Yemm*	3.00
_____ NATURE'S MEDICINES *Richard Lucas*	3.00
_____ VEGETABLE GARDENING FOR BEGINNERS *Hugh Wiberg*	2.00
_____ VEGETABLES FOR TODAY'S GARDENS *R. Milton Carleton*	2.00
_____ VEGETARIAN COOKERY *Janet Walker*	4.00
_____ VEGETARIAN COOKING MADE EASY & DELECTABLE *Veronica Vezza*	3.00
_____ VEGETARIAN DELIGHTS—A Happy Cookbook for Health *K. R. Mehta*	2.00
_____ VEGETARIAN GOURMET COOKBOOK *Joyce McKinnel*	3.00

GAMBLING & POKER

_____ ADVANCED POKER STRATEGY & WINNING PLAY *A. D. Livingston*	5.00
_____ HOW NOT TO LOSE AT POKER *Jeffrey Lloyd Castle*	3.00
_____ HOW TO WIN AT DICE GAMES *Skip Frey*	3.00
_____ HOW TO WIN AT POKER *Terence Reese & Anthony T. Watkins*	5.00
_____ WINNING AT CRAPS *Dr. Lloyd T. Commins*	4.00
_____ WINNING AT GIN *Chester Wander & Cy Rice*	3.00
_____ WINNING AT POKER—An Expert's Guide *John Archer*	5.00
_____ WINNING AT 21—An Expert's Guide *John Archer*	5.00
_____ WINNING POKER SYSTEMS *Norman Zadeh*	3.00

HEALTH

_____ BEE POLLEN *Lynda Lyngheim & Jack Scagnetti*	3.00
_____ DR. LINDNER'S SPECIAL WEIGHT CONTROL METHOD *P. G. Lindner, M.D.*	2.00
_____ HELP YOURSELF TO BETTER SIGHT *Margaret Darst Corbett*	3.00
_____ HOW TO IMPROVE YOUR VISION *Dr. Robert A. Kraskin*	3.00
_____ HOW YOU CAN STOP SMOKING PERMANENTLY *Ernest Caldwell*	3.00
_____ MIND OVER PLATTER *Peter G. Lindner, M.D.*	3.00
_____ NATURE'S WAY TO NUTRITION & VIBRANT HEALTH *Robert J. Scrutton*	3.00
_____ NEW CARBOHYDRATE DIET COUNTER *Patti Lopez-Pereira*	2.00
_____ QUICK & EASY EXERCISES FOR FACIAL BEAUTY *Judy Smith-deal*	2.00
_____ QUICK & EASY EXERCISES FOR FIGURE BEAUTY *Judy Smith-deal*	2.00
_____ REFLEXOLOGY *Dr. Maybelle Segal*	3.00
_____ REFLEXOLOGY FOR GOOD HEALTH *Anna Kaye & Don C. Matchan*	4.00
_____ 30 DAYS TO BEAUTIFUL LEGS *Dr. Marc Selner*	3.00
_____ YOU CAN LEARN TO RELAX *Dr. Samuel Gutwirth*	3.00
_____ YOUR ALLERGY—What To Do About It *Allan Knight, M.D.*	3.00

HOBBIES

_____ BEACHCOMBING FOR BEGINNERS *Norman Hickin*	2.00
_____ BLACKSTONE'S MODERN CARD TRICKS *Harry Blackstone*	3.00
_____ BLACKSTONE'S SECRETS OF MAGIC *Harry Blackstone*	3.00
_____ COIN COLLECTING FOR BEGINNERS *Burton Hobson & Fred Reinfeld*	3.00
_____ ENTERTAINING WITH ESP *Tony 'Doc' Shiels*	2.00
_____ 400 FASCINATING MAGIC TRICKS YOU CAN DO *Howard Thurston*	4.00
_____ HOW I TURN JUNK INTO FUN AND PROFIT *Sari*	3.00
_____ HOW TO WRITE A HIT SONG & SELL IT *Tommy Boyce*	7.00
_____ JUGGLING MADE EASY *Rudolf Dittrich*	3.00
_____ MAGIC FOR ALL AGES *Walter Gibson*	4.00
_____ MAGIC MADE EASY *Byron Wels*	2.00
_____ STAMP COLLECTING FOR BEGINNERS *Burton Hobson*	3.00

HORSE PLAYERS' WINNING GUIDES

_____ BETTING HORSES TO WIN *Les Conklin*	3.00
_____ ELIMINATE THE LOSERS *Bob McKnight*	3.00
_____ HOW TO PICK WINNING HORSES *Bob McKnight*	5.00

____ HOW TO WIN AT THE RACES *Sam (The Genius) Lewin*		5.00
____ HOW YOU CAN BEAT THE RACES *Jack Kavanagh*		5.00
____ MAKING MONEY AT THE RACES *David Barr*		3.00
____ PAYDAY AT THE RACES *Les Conklin*		3.00
____ SMART HANDICAPPING MADE EASY *William Bauman*		5.00
____ SUCCESS AT THE HARNESS RACES *Barry Meadow*		5.00
____ WINNING AT THE HARNESS RACES—An Expert's Guide *Nick Cammarano*		5.00

HUMOR

____ HOW TO BE A COMEDIAN FOR FUN & PROFIT *King & Laufer*		2.00
____ HOW TO FLATTEN YOUR TUSH *Coach Marge Reardon*		2.00
____ HOW TO MAKE LOVE TO YOURSELF *Ron Stevens & Joy Grdnic*		3.00
____ JOKE TELLER'S HANDBOOK *Bob Orben*		4.00
____ JOKES FOR ALL OCCASIONS *Al Schock*		4.00
____ 2000 NEW LAUGHS FOR SPEAKERS *Bob Orben*		5.00
____ 2,500 JOKES TO START 'EM LAUGHING *Bob Orben*		5.00

HYPNOTISM

____ ADVANCED TECHNIQUES OF HYPNOSIS *Melvin Powers*		3.00
____ BRAINWASHING AND THE CULTS *Paul A. Verdier, Ph.D.*		3.00
____ CHILDBIRTH WITH HYPNOSIS *William S. Kroger, M.D.*		5.00
____ HOW TO SOLVE Your Sex Problems with Self-Hypnosis *Frank S. Caprio, M.D.*		5.00
____ HOW TO STOP SMOKING THRU SELF-HYPNOSIS *Leslie M. LeCron*		3.00
____ HOW TO USE AUTO-SUGGESTION EFFECTIVELY *John Duckworth*		3.00
____ HOW YOU CAN BOWL BETTER USING SELF-HYPNOSIS *Jack Heise*		3.00
____ HOW YOU CAN PLAY BETTER GOLF USING SELF-HYPNOSIS *Jack Heise*		3.00
____ HYPNOSIS AND SELF-HYPNOSIS *Bernard Hollander, M.D.*		3.00
____ HYPNOTISM *(Originally published in 1893) Carl Sextus*		5.00
____ HYPNOTISM & PSYCHIC PHENOMENA *Simeon Edmunds*		4.00
____ HYPNOTISM MADE EASY *Dr. Ralph Winn*		5.00
____ HYPNOTISM MADE PRACTICAL *Louis Orton*		5.00
____ HYPNOTISM REVEALED *Melvin Powers*		2.00
____ HYPNOTISM TODAY *Leslie LeCron and Jean Bordeaux, Ph.D.*		5.00
____ MODERN HYPNOSIS *Lesley Kuhn & Salvatore Russo, Ph.D.*		5.00
____ NEW CONCEPTS OF HYPNOSIS *Bernard C. Gindes, M.D.*		5.00
____ NEW SELF-HYPNOSIS *Paul Adams*		5.00
____ POST-HYPNOTIC INSTRUCTIONS—Suggestions for Therapy *Arnold Furst*		5.00
____ PRACTICAL GUIDE TO SELF-HYPNOSIS *Melvin Powers*		3.00
____ PRACTICAL HYPNOTISM *Philip Magonet, M.D.*		3.00
____ SECRETS OF HYPNOTISM *S. J. Van Pelt, M.D.*		5.00
____ SELF-HYPNOSIS A Conditioned-Response Technique *Laurence Sparks*		5.00
____ SELF-HYPNOSIS Its Theory, Technique & Application *Melvin Powers*		3.00
____ THERAPY THROUGH HYPNOSIS *edited by Raphael H. Rhodes*		4.00

JUDAICA

____ MODERN ISRAEL *Lily Edelman*		2.00
____ SERVICE OF THE HEART *Evelyn Garfiel, Ph.D.*		4.00
____ STORY OF ISRAEL IN COINS *Jean & Maurice Gould*		2.00
____ STORY OF ISRAEL IN STAMPS *Maxim & Gabriel Shamir*		1.00
____ TONGUE OF THE PROPHETS *Robert St. John*		5.00

JUST FOR WOMEN

____ COSMOPOLITAN'S GUIDE TO MARVELOUS MEN Fwd. by *Helen Gurley Brown*		3.00
____ COSMOPOLITAN'S HANG-UP HANDBOOK Foreword by *Helen Gurley Brown*		4.00
____ COSMOPOLITAN'S LOVE BOOK—A Guide to Ecstasy in Bed		5.00
____ COSMOPOLITAN'S NEW ETIQUETTE GUIDE Fwd. by *Helen Gurley Brown*		4.00
____ I AM A COMPLEAT WOMAN *Doris Hagopian & Karen O'Connor Sweeney*		3.00
____ JUST FOR WOMEN—A Guide to the Female Body *Richard E. Sand, M.D.*		5.00
____ NEW APPROACHES TO SEX IN MARRIAGE *John E. Eichenlaub, M.D.*		3.00
____ SEXUALLY ADEQUATE FEMALE *Frank S. Caprio, M.D.*		3.00
____ SEXUALLY FULFILLED WOMAN *Dr. Rachel Copelan*		5.00
____ YOUR FIRST YEAR OF MARRIAGE *Dr. Tom McGinnis*		3.00

MARRIAGE, SEX & PARENTHOOD

____ ABILITY TO LOVE *Dr. Allan Fromme*		6.00

____ GUIDE TO SUCCESSFUL MARRIAGE *Drs. Albert Ellis & Robert Harper*		5.00
____ HOW TO RAISE AN EMOTIONALLY HEALTHY, HAPPY CHILD *A. Ellis*		4.00
____ SEX WITHOUT GUILT *Albert Ellis, Ph.D.*		5.00
____ SEXUALLY ADEQUATE MALE *Frank S. Caprio, M.D.*		3.00
____ SEXUALLY FULFILLED MAN *Dr. Rachel Copelan*		5.00

MELVIN POWERS' MAIL ORDER LIBRARY

____ HOW TO GET RICH IN MAIL ORDER *Melvin Powers*		15.00
____ HOW TO WRITE A GOOD ADVERTISEMENT *Victor O. Schwab*		15.00
____ MAIL ORDER MADE EASY *J. Frank Brumbaugh*		10.00
____ U.S. MAIL ORDER SHOPPER'S GUIDE *Susan Spitzer*		10.00

METAPHYSICS & OCCULT

____ BOOK OF TALISMANS, AMULETS & ZODIACAL GEMS *William Pavitt*		5.00
____ CONCENTRATION—A Guide to Mental Mastery *Mouni Sadhu*		5.00
____ CRITIQUES OF GOD *Edited by Peter Angeles*		7.00
____ EXTRA-TERRESTRIAL INTELLIGENCE—The First Encounter		6.00
____ FORTUNE TELLING WITH CARDS *P. Foli*		4.00
____ HANDWRITING ANALYSIS MADE EASY *John Marley*		4.00
____ HANDWRITING TELLS *Nadya Olyanova*		5.00
____ HOW TO INTERPRET DREAMS, OMENS & FORTUNE TELLING SIGNS *Gettings*		3.00
____ HOW TO UNDERSTAND YOUR DREAMS *Geoffrey A. Dudley*		3.00
____ ILLUSTRATED YOGA *William Zorn*		3.00
____ IN DAYS OF GREAT PEACE *Mouni Sadhu*		3.00
____ LSD—THE AGE OF MIND *Bernard Roseman*		2.00
____ MAGICIAN—His Training and Work *W. E. Butler*		3.00
____ MEDITATION *Mouni Sadhu*		7.00
____ MODERN NUMEROLOGY *Morris C. Goodman*		3.00
____ NUMEROLOGY—ITS FACTS AND SECRETS *Ariel Yvon Taylor*		3.00
____ NUMEROLOGY MADE EASY *W. Mykian*		4.00
____ PALMISTRY MADE EASY *Fred Gettings*		5.00
____ PALMISTRY MADE PRACTICAL *Elizabeth Daniels Squire*		4.00
____ PALMISTRY SECRETS REVEALED *Henry Frith*		3.00
____ PROPHECY IN OUR TIME *Martin Ebon*		2.50
____ PSYCHOLOGY OF HANDWRITING *Nadya Olyanova*		5.00
____ SUPERSTITION—Are You Superstitious? *Eric Maple*		2.00
____ TAROT *Mouni Sadhu*		8.00
____ TAROT OF THE BOHEMIANS *Papus*		5.00
____ WAYS TO SELF-REALIZATION *Mouni Sadhu*		3.00
____ WHAT YOUR HANDWRITING REVEALS *Albert E. Hughes*		3.00
____ WITCHCRAFT, MAGIC & OCCULTISM—A Fascinating History *W. B. Crow*		5.00
____ WITCHCRAFT—THE SIXTH SENSE *Justine Glass*		5.00
____ WORLD OF PSYCHIC RESEARCH *Hereward Carrington*		2.00

SELF-HELP & INSPIRATIONAL

____ DAILY POWER FOR JOYFUL LIVING *Dr. Donald Curtis*		5.00
____ DYNAMIC THINKING *Melvin Powers*		2.00
____ GREATEST POWER IN THE UNIVERSE *U. S. Andersen*		5.00
____ GROW RICH WHILE YOU SLEEP *Ben Sweetland*		3.00
____ GROWTH THROUGH REASON *Albert Ellis, Ph.D.*		4.00
____ GUIDE TO PERSONAL HAPPINESS *Albert Ellis, Ph.D. & Irving Becker, Ed. D.*		5.00
____ HELPING YOURSELF WITH APPLIED PSYCHOLOGY *R. Henderson*		2.00
____ HOW TO ATTRACT GOOD LUCK *A. H. Z. Carr*		5.00
____ HOW TO DEVELOP A WINNING PERSONALITY *Martin Panzer*		5.00
____ HOW TO DEVELOP AN EXCEPTIONAL MEMORY *Young & Gibson*		5.00
____ HOW TO LIVE WITH A NEUROTIC *Albert Ellis, Ph. D.*		5.00
____ HOW TO OVERCOME YOUR FEARS *M. P. Leahy, M.D.*		3.00
____ HOW YOU CAN HAVE CONFIDENCE AND POWER *Les Giblin*		5.00
____ HUMAN PROBLEMS & HOW TO SOLVE THEM *Dr. Donald Curtis*		5.00
____ I CAN *Ben Sweetland*		5.00
____ I WILL *Ben Sweetland*		3.00
____ LEFT-HANDED PEOPLE *Michael Barsley*		5.00
____ MAGIC IN YOUR MIND *U. S. Andersen*		6.00
____ MAGIC OF THINKING BIG *Dr. David J. Schwartz*		3.00

____ MAGIC POWER OF YOUR MIND *Walter M. Germain*		5.00
____ MENTAL POWER THROUGH SLEEP SUGGESTION *Melvin Powers*		3.00
____ NEW GUIDE TO RATIONAL LIVING *Albert Ellis, Ph.D. & R. Harper, Ph.D.*		3.00
____ PROJECT YOU *A Manual of Rational Assertiveness Training Paris & Casey*		6.00
____ PSYCHO-CYBERNETICS *Maxwell Maltz, M.D.*		5.00
____ SCIENCE OF MIND IN DAILY LIVING *Dr. Donald Curtis*		5.00
____ SECRET OF SECRETS *U. S. Andersen*		6.00
____ SECRET POWER OF THE PYRAMIDS *U. S. Andersen*		5.00
____ STUTTERING AND WHAT YOU CAN DO ABOUT IT *W. Johnson, Ph.D.*		2.50
____ SUCCESS-CYBERNETICS *U. S. Andersen*		6.00
____ 10 DAYS TO A GREAT NEW LIFE *William E. Edwards*		3.00
____ THINK AND GROW RICH *Napoleon Hill*		5.00
____ THINK YOUR WAY TO SUCCESS *Dr. Lew Losoncy*		5.00
____ THREE MAGIC WORDS *U. S. Andersen*		5.00
____ TREASURY OF COMFORT *edited by Rabbi Sidney Greenberg*		5.00
____ TREASURY OF THE ART OF LIVING *Sidney S. Greenberg*		5.00
____ YOU ARE NOT THE TARGET *Laura Huxley*		5.00
____ YOUR SUBCONSCIOUS POWER *Charles M. Simmons*		5.00
____ YOUR THOUGHTS CAN CHANGE YOUR LIFE *Dr. Donald Curtis*		5.00

SPORTS

____ BICYCLING FOR FUN AND GOOD HEALTH *Kenneth E. Luther*		2.00
____ BILLIARDS—Pocket • Carom • Three Cushion *Clive Cottingham, Jr.*		3.00
____ CAMPING-OUT 101 Ideas & Activities *Bruno Knobel*		2.00
____ COMPLETE GUIDE TO FISHING *Vlad Evanoff*		2.00
____ HOW TO IMPROVE YOUR RACQUETBALL *Lubarsky Kaufman & Scagnetti*		3.00
____ HOW TO WIN AT POCKET BILLIARDS *Edward D. Knuchell*		5.00
____ JOY OF WALKING *Jack Scagnetti*		3.00
____ LEARNING & TEACHING SOCCER SKILLS *Eric Worthington*		3.00
____ MOTORCYCLING FOR BEGINNERS *I. G. Edmonds*		3.00
____ RACQUETBALL FOR WOMEN *Toni Hudson, Jack Scagnetti & Vince Rondone*		3.00
____ RACQUETBALL MADE EASY *Steve Lubarsky, Rod Delson & Jack Scagnetti*		4.00
____ SECRET OF BOWLING STRIKES *Dawson Taylor*		3.00
____ SECRET OF PERFECT PUTTING *Horton Smith & Dawson Taylor*		3.00
____ SOCCER—The Game & How to Play It *Gary Rosenthal*		3.00
____ STARTING SOCCER *Edward F. Dolan, Jr.*		3.00

TENNIS LOVERS' LIBRARY

____ BEGINNER'S GUIDE TO WINNING TENNIS *Helen Hull Jacobs*		2.00
____ HOW TO BEAT BETTER TENNIS PLAYERS *Loring Fiske*		4.00
____ HOW TO IMPROVE YOUR TENNIS—Style, Strategy & Analysis *C. Wilson*		2.00
____ INSIDE TENNIS—Techniques of Winning *Jim Leighton*		3.00
____ PLAY TENNIS WITH ROSEWALL *Ken Rosewall*		2.00
____ PSYCH YOURSELF TO BETTER TENNIS *Dr. Walter A. Luszki*		2.00
____ TENNIS FOR BEGINNERS, *Dr. H. A. Murray*		2.00
____ TENNIS MADE EASY *Joel Brecheen*		4.00
____ WEEKEND TENNIS—How to Have Fun & Win at the Same Time *Bill Talbert*		3.00
____ WINNING WITH PERCENTAGE TENNIS—Smart Strategy *Jack Lowe*		2.00

WILSHIRE PET LIBRARY

____ DOG OBEDIENCE TRAINING *Gust Kessopulos*		5.00
____ DOG TRAINING MADE EASY & FUN *John W. Kellogg*		4.00
____ HOW TO BRING UP YOUR PET DOG *Kurt Unkelbach*		2.00
____ HOW TO RAISE & TRAIN YOUR PUPPY *Jeff Griffen*		3.00
____ PIGEONS: HOW TO RAISE & TRAIN THEM *William H. Allen, Jr.*		2.00

*The books listed above can be obtained from your book dealer or directly from
Melvin Powers. When ordering, please remit 50¢ per book postage & handling.
Send for our free illustrated catalog of self-improvement books.*

Melvin Powers
12015 Sherman Road, No. Hollywood, California 91605

WILSHIRE HORSE LOVERS' LIBRARY

____ AMATEUR HORSE BREEDER *A. C. Leighton Hardman*	5.00
____ AMERICAN QUARTER HORSE IN PICTURES *Margaret Cabell Self*	3.00
____ APPALOOSA HORSE *Donna & Bill Richardson*	5.00
____ ARABIAN HORSE *Reginald S. Summerhays*	4.00
____ ART OF WESTERN RIDING *Suzanne Norton Jones*	5.00
____ AT THE HORSE SHOW *Margaret Cabell Self*	3.00
____ BACK-YARD HORSE *Peggy Jett Pittinger*	4.00
____ BASIC DRESSAGE *Jean Froissard*	5.00
____ BEGINNER'S GUIDE TO HORSEBACK RIDING *Sheila Wall*	2.00
____ BEGINNER'S GUIDE TO THE WESTERN HORSE *Natlee Kenoyer*	2.00
____ BITS—THEIR HISTORY, USE AND MISUSE *Louis Taylor*	5.00
____ BREAKING & TRAINING THE DRIVING HORSE *Doris Ganton*	10.00
____ BREAKING YOUR HORSE'S BAD HABITS *W. Dayton Sumner*	5.00
____ COMPLETE TRAINING OF HORSE AND RIDER *Colonel Alois Podhajsky*	6.00
____ DISORDERS OF THE HORSE & WHAT TO DO ABOUT THEM *E. Hanauer*	5.00
____ DOG TRAINING MADE EASY & FUN *John W. Kellogg*	4.00
____ DRESSAGE—A Study of the Finer Points in Riding *Henry Wynmalen*	5.00
____ DRIVE ON *Doris Ganton*	7.00
____ DRIVING HORSES *Sallie Walrond*	5.00
____ EQUITATION *Jean Froissard*	5.00
____ FIRST AID FOR HORSES *Dr. Charles H. Denning, Jr.*	3.00
____ FUN OF RAISING A COLT *Rubye & Frank Griffith*	5.00
____ FUN ON HORSEBACK *Margaret Caball Self*	4.00
____ GYMKHANA GAMES *Natlee Kenoyer*	2.00
____ HORSE DISEASES—Causes, Symptoms & Treatment *Dr. H. G. Belschner*	6.00
____ HORSE OWNER'S CONCISE GUIDE *Elsie V. Hanauer*	3.00
____ HORSE SELECTION & CARE FOR BEGINNERS *George H. Conn*	5.00
____ HORSEBACK RIDING FOR BEGINNERS *Louis Taylor*	5.00
____ HORSEBACK RIDING MADE EASY & FUN *Sue Henderson Coen*	5.00
____ HORSES—Their Selection, Care & Handling *Margaret Cabell Self*	5.00
____ HOW TO BUY A BETTER HORSE & SELL THE HORSE YOU OWN	3.00
____ HOW TO ENJOY YOUR QUARTER HORSE *Willard H. Porter*	3.00
____ HUNTER IN PICTURES *Margaret Cabell Self*	2.00
____ ILLUSTRATED BOOK OF THE HORSE *S. Sidney* (8½″ × 11″)	10.00
____ ILLUSTRATED HORSE MANAGEMENT—400 Illustrations *Dr. E. Mayhew*	6.00
____ ILLUSTRATED HORSE TRAINING *Captain M. H. Hayes*	5.00
____ ILLUSTRATED HORSEBACK RIDING FOR BEGINNERS *Jeanne Mellin*	3.00
____ JUMPING—Learning & Teaching *Jean Froissard*	5.00
____ KNOW ALL ABOUT HORSES *Harry Disston*	3.00
____ LAME HORSE Cause, Symptoms & Treatment *Dr. James R. Rooney*	5.00
____ LAW & YOUR HORSE *Edward H. Greene*	7.00
____ MANUAL OF HORSEMANSHIP *Harold Black*	5.00
____ MOVIE HORSES—The Fascinating Techniques of Training *Anthony Amaral*	2.00
____ POLICE HORSES *Judith Campbell*	2.00
____ PRACTICAL GUIDE TO HORSESHOEING	5.00
____ PRACTICAL GUIDE TO OWNING YOUR OWN HORSE *Steven D. Price*	3.00
____ PRACTICAL HORSE PSYCHOLOGY *Moyra Williams*	4.00
____ PROBLEM HORSES Guide for Curing Serious Behavior Habits *Summerhays*	4.00
____ REINSMAN OF THE WEST—BRIDLES & BITS *Ed Connell*	5.00
____ RESCHOOLING THE THOROUGHBRED *Peggy Jett Pittenger*	3.00
____ RIDE WESTERN *Louis Taylor*	5.00
____ SCHOOLING YOUR YOUNG HORSE *George Wheatley*	5.00
____ STABLE MANAGEMENT FOR THE OWNER-GROOM *George Wheatley*	4.00
____ STALLION MANAGEMENT—A Guide for Stud Owners *A. C. Hardman*	5.00
____ TEACHING YOUR HORSE TO JUMP *W. J. Froud*	2.00
____ TRAINING YOUR HORSE TO SHOW *Neale Haley*	5.00
____ TREATING COMMON DISEASES OF YOUR HORSE *Dr. George H. Conn*	5.00
____ TREATING HORSE AILMENTS *G. W. Serth*	2.00
____ YOU AND YOUR PONY *Pepper Mainwaring Healey* (8½″ × 11″)	6.00
____ YOUR FIRST HORSE *George C. Saunders, M.D.*	5.00
____ YOUR PONY BOOK *Hermann Wiederhold*	2.00

*The books listed above can be obtained from your book dealer or directly from
Melvin Powers. When ordering, please remit 50ᶜ per book postage & handling.
Send for our free illustrated catalog of self-improvement books.*

Melvin Powers
12015 Sherman Road, No. Hollywood, California 91605

Notes

Notes